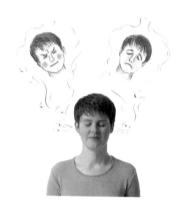

HEALTH AND HEALING
THE NATURAL WAY

# MANAGING
# PAIN

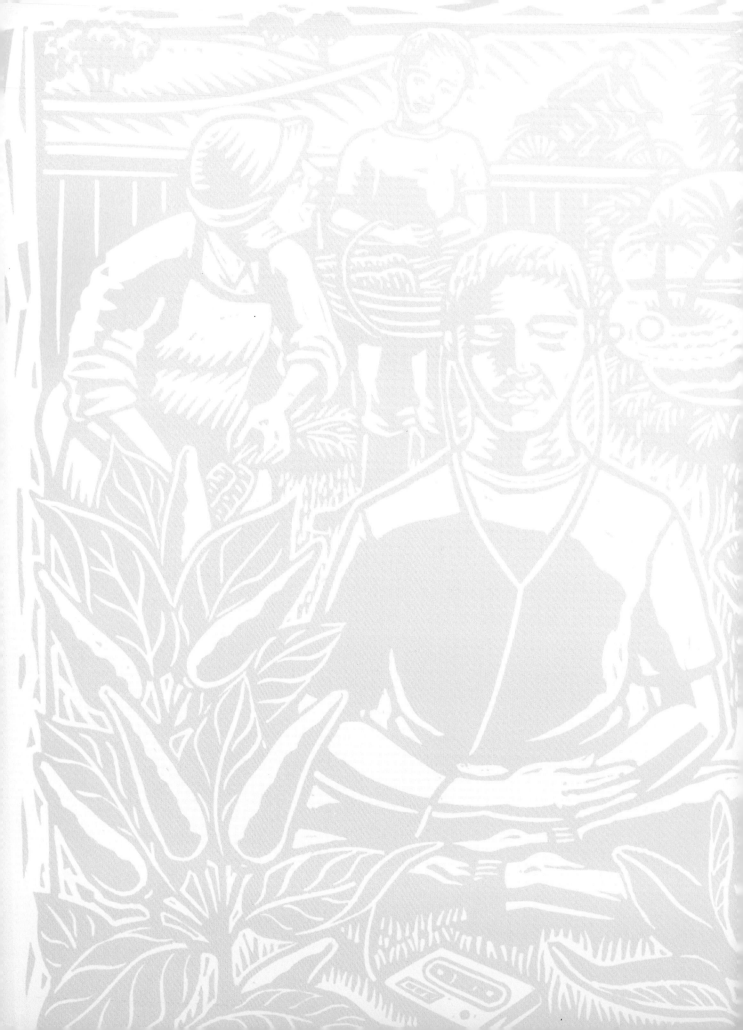

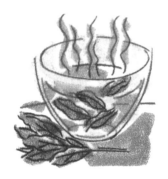

*Health And Healing*
*The Natural Way*

# Managing
# Pain

Published by
The Reader's Digest Association Limited
London New York Sydney Montreal Cape Town

MANAGING PAIN
was created and produced by
Carroll & Brown Limited
5 Lonsdale Road, London NW6 6RA
for The Reader's Digest Association Limited, London

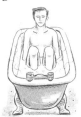

### CARROLL & BROWN

**Publishing Director** Denis Kennedy
**Art Director** Chrissie Lloyd

**Managing Editor** Sandra Rigby
**Managing Art Editor** Tracy Timson

**Editors** Richard Emerson, Hilary Sagar

**Art Editor** Simon Daley
**Designer** Jonathan Wainwright

**Photographers** Jules Selmes, David Murray

**Production** Christine Corton, Wendy Rogers

**Computer Management** John Clifford, Karen Kloot

First English Edition Copyright © 1997
The Reader's Digest Association Limited,
11 Westferry Circus, Canary Wharf,
London E14 4HE

Copyright © 1997
The Reader's Digest Association Far East Limited
Philippines Copyright © 1997
The Reader's Digest Association Far East Limited

ISBN 0 276 42265 1

Reproduced by Colourscan, Singapore
Printing and binding: Printer Industria Gráfica S.A., Barcelona

### MEDICAL CONSULTANT

Dr J.R. Wiles, MB, BS(Lond), FRCA
*Director of the Centre for Pain Relief, The Walton Centre for
Neurology & Neurosurgery, Liverpool, UK*

### COMPLEMENTARY HEALTH CONSULTANT

Michael Endacott
*Research Director, The Institute for
Complementary Medicine, London, UK*

### CONTRIBUTORS

Dr E. Ghadiali, BSc, MPsychol, PhD, CPsychol, AFBPsS
*Consultant Clinical Neuropsychologist*

Dr Andrew Baronowski, BSc Hons, MB BS, MD, FRCA
*Consultant in Pain Management*

Dr Tim Nash MBBS, DObstRCOG, FRCA
*Consultant in Pain Relief*

Dr Turo Nurmikko, MD, PHD
*Consultant in Pain Management*

Roger Newman-Turner BAc, ND, DO, MRO, MRN
*Registered naturopath, osteopath and acupuncturist*

Rosalie Everatt, RGN
*Founder of Pain Concern UK and Pain Wise UK*

Professor Philip-John Lamey,
BSc, BDS, MBChB, DDS, FDS, RCPS, FFD, RCSI
*Professor of Oral Medicine*

H.P.J. Walsh Mch.Orth, FRCS
*Consultant Orthopaedic Surgeon*

#### FOR THE READER'S DIGEST

**Series Editor** Christine Noble
**Editorial Assistant** Alison Candlin

#### READER'S DIGEST GENERAL BOOKS

**Editorial Director** Cortina Butler
**Art Director** Nick Clark

The information in this book is for reference only;
it is not intended as a substitute for a doctor's diagnosis and care.
The editors urge anyone with continuing medical problems
or symptoms to consult a doctor.

# MANAGING PAIN

More and more people today are choosing to take greater responsibility for their own health rather than relying on the doctor to step in with a cure when something goes wrong. We now recognise that we can influence our health by making an improvement in lifestyle – a better diet, more exercise and reduced stress. People are also becoming increasingly aware that there are other healing methods – some new, others very ancient – that can help to prevent illness or be used as a complement to orthodox medicine.

The series *Health and Healing the Natural Way* will help you to make your own health choices by giving you clear, comprehensive, straightforward and encouraging information and advice about methods of improving your health. The series explains the many different natural therapies now available – aromatherapy, herbalism, acupressure and many others – and the circumstances in which they may be of benefit when used in conjunction with conventional medicine.

A lack of information about the nature of pain and its causes can often lead to fear – the greatest barrier to the control of painful symptoms. *MANAGING PAIN* aims to fill this knowledge gap with clear and practical information to help banish that fear. It explains the positive role that the pain response plays in the functioning of the body, and shows how pain can be relieved or controlled by self-help measures, changes in lifestyle and, where necessary, by finding the most suitable treatment for your needs. While conventional painkillers have a part to play in pain control, they can never provide a complete answer. In particular, in the case of persistent or recurrent pain, they can lead to negative patterns of behaviour in which pain and medication come to dominate your life. In *MANAGING PAIN* we show that appropriate measures, coupled with a positive approach, can enable you to regain control of your body and life, and enhance your health and well-being.

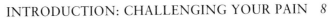

# CONTENTS

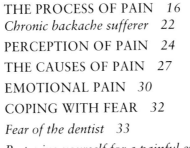
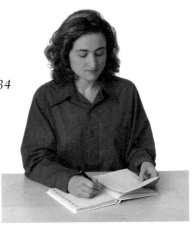

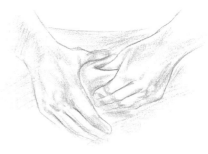

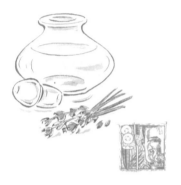

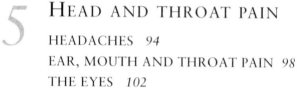

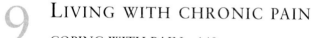
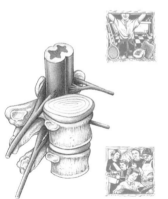

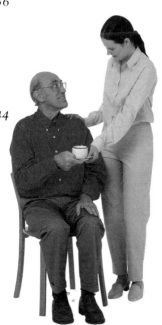

# CHALLENGING YOUR PAIN

*Pain, particularly chronic pain, is one of the most debilitating of conditions, yet there are steps you can take to avoid, minimise or relieve pain altogether.*

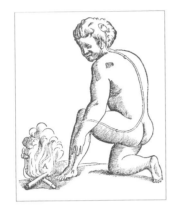

**THE PATH OF PAIN**
*The philosopher Descartes was one of the first people to describe the passage of pain messages to the brain. He envisaged a message travelling from the site of the injury up the body to trigger an alarm response in the brain.*

**NATURAL PAIN CONTROL**
*Many herbal remedies, such as camomile tea, date back thousands of years and can still be used effectively today in the treatment of various painful afflictions.*

Pain often produces dependence on doctors and drugs. People tend to expect the doctor to wave a magic wand and take pain away, and over 80 per cent of the population in the United Kingdom take painkillers on a regular basis. But painkillers don't provide an answer to pain, especially in the long term. In fact, there is no easy solution: increasingly we are learning that successful pain management for chronic pain requires the active involvement of individual sufferers, so that they gain an understanding of their pain – and ultimately take responsibility for controlling it. This book aims to describe the mechanics of pain, how it works and what feeds it, and thus provide a key to effective pain management.

## PAIN AND WESTERN MEDICINE

The traditional approach of Western medicine to pain management has tended to focus on blocking the experience of pain by chemical means. As recently as 1842 surgeons could only use alcohol as a painkiller. Morphine was used during the American Civil War, but the problem of addiction made its widespread use undesirable. In 1847 chloroform was first administered to relieve labour pains and was soon in use during a range of surgical procedures, but high levels of the chemical proved to cause liver damage. It was only in the 1930s that anaesthesia became a relatively safe practice.

Conventional medicine is still likely to be the first 'port of call' for the majority of pain sufferers. But many people feel that modern medicine is still too focused on drug therapy and does not allow patients a sufficiently active part in the management of their conditions. In addition, Western medicine has had only limited success in managing complex pain problems. Chronic pain conditions such as arthritis or backache tend not to respond well to conventional treatment. Now many people are taking an interest in therapies that tackle pain in a different way. These methods offer patients a choice, but can also be used to complement conventional treatment.

## PAIN RELIEF IN OTHER CULTURES

Although individual techniques differ, many Eastern systems of medicine share a focus in looking at patients' particular pain problems within the context of their overall general health and issues of diet, lifestyle and emotional well-being. For example, traditional Chinese medicine incorporates a range of treatments such as acupuncture, herbalism, massage, diet control and exercise, all based on the general philosophy that good health revolves round the correct flow of *chi*, the body's energy. Although Western science has been sceptical of the principles behind Chinese medicine, many practitioners are now becoming convinced of the efficacy of acupuncture and Chinese herbs in the treatment of a range of pain problems including backache, muscular and joint pain, migraines and period pain.

Similarly Ayurveda, the traditional medicine of India, is another complete philosophy of health based on energy balance. As well as placing great importance on diet and lifestyle, it emphasises massage and meditation. Today many Western practitioners recognise that such techniques, which promote relaxation and reduce stress, can help people to cope better with pain. Many pain clinics offer a range of treatment methods from counselling to aromatherapy that can help the patient to learn to relax.

## THE HOLISTIC APPROACH TO PAIN

Increasingly modern science is recognising what traditional medical systems have practised for centuries: effective pain management must be holistic, addressing the lifestyle and emotional and spiritual health of the patient, as well as the physical problem. Recent research has proven that our perception of pain is controlled

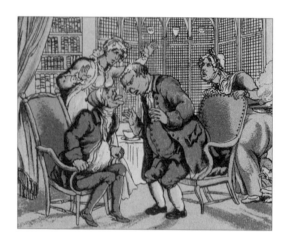

*EARLY WESTERN MEDICINE*
*Until the early 19th century, Western medicine was based on limited scientific knowledge and a poor understanding of the body. Physicians were often lampooned in cartoons, such as this 1812 example by Thomas Rowlandson from his famous 'Dr Syntax' series.*

*MIND OVER PAIN*
*Eastern therapists take a holistic or 'whole body' approach to pain. Yoga, for example, enables some people to strengthen the link between mind and body and so control pain impulses.*

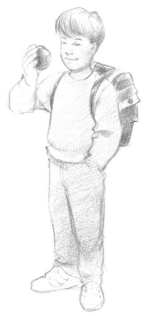

**POSTURE AND PAIN**
*Recent research has shown the importance of good posture in preventing the onset of back pain. Carrying a backpack is better for your posture than carrying a satchel or a suitcase, for example.*

**DIET AND PAIN**
*A balanced diet that includes plenty of fresh vegetables and fruit not only helps to ward off many painful disorders but may also help those with chronic conditions to control their pain.*

by a whole range of factors: the experience of pain is a highly individualistic one and is affected not only by a person's state of health, but also by age, cultural background and emotions.

Although most people find it easy to grasp the concept that general health can influence their pain, it is only relatively recently that doctors have begun to address diet and exercise as part of an overall pain management plan. Yet many kinds of pain can be avoided or relieved by simple lifestyle changes. For instance, reducing fat intake can have an impact on the pain of angina, lower the risk of some types of cancer, and reduce body weight, thereby decreasing the pain of disorders such as arthritis. Exercise is just as important in both preventing and relieving pain. It was once believed that people with chronic back pain should rest until they recovered, even if it took years. It is now known that both acute and chronic back pain benefit from regular moderate exercise. Moreover, exercise plays a vital role in preventing painful diseases such as osteoporosis and heart disease, as well as the painful stiffness that often comes with ageing.

People are even less well-informed about the very real role played by stress and the emotions in pain. Science has now found evidence to show how prolonged stress reduces the body's own natural painkillers, endorphins, and makes the experience of pain more severe. A state of stress causes direct physical changes in the body; the muscles tense, which in turn aggravates the pain experienced in such conditions as backache. Stress relief measures can play a large part in overcoming the anxiety and depression experienced by many sufferers of chronic pain. For this reason relaxation and meditation therapies are proving increasingly valuable in helping people with long-term pain.

## UNDERSTANDING PAIN

While a great deal is being learnt from traditional forms of medicine, modern science has also revealed much about the workings of the nervous system and the brain, and how this affects the perception of pain. What is becoming increasingly clear is that there are steps that an individual can take to control his or her perception of pain messages. Understanding pain and how it works enables you to take these steps to avoid the pain or to minimise it. Pain is usually meaningful: it is your body's way of warning you that you have injured yourself, or that you are about to come to harm, or that you need to rest. All pain sensations are processed in the brain. Your brain will decide what a pain message means, how serious it is, and the most appropriate action to take. In the case of a cut finger, for example, the pain message effectively forces you to rest the injured part in order to avoid further damage and allow the body's natural healing processes to take place. However, in the case of chronic pain, the pain message is not a useful one. Arthritis is in fact made worse by rest, yet the pain experienced by the sufferer when he or she tries to become more mobile discourages any kind of exercise at all.

Pain research is now focusing on how individuals can influence the way the brain deals with information received from the nervous system. For example, studies have shown that when an individual is experiencing moments of extreme stress, such as an athlete taking part in a major competition, quite serious injuries can be sustained without the person being aware of the injury until the event is over. The brain has decided that the event is more important than the pain. In the case of chronic pain it might be possible to refocus the brain so that instead of prioritising, say, a persistent message of back pain, it decides that completing a 20 minute daily exercise programme is more important and overrides the pain message.

## THE BEST TREATMENT FOR YOUR PAIN

No pain experience is straightforward, and each individual's experience of pain is unique. It follows that finding the best therapy is a highly individualistic process. In some cases, orthodox medicine such as surgery may be necessary, but in other cases you might seek help from a naturopath for advice on diet and herbal remedies, an osteopath for back and neck manipulation, an acupuncturist for pain relief, or combine a range of treatments to best manage your pain. The key to success is understanding how pain messages are processed so you feel in control of your pain, rather than ruled by it.

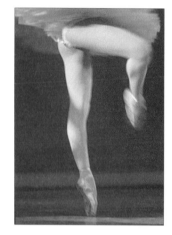

*THE STRENGTH TO ENDURE*
*Dancers provide an ideal example of how the mind can control pain. As they strive to achieve perfect form and movement, ballerinas endure great pain – and rise above it.*

*WHERE EAST MEETS WEST*
*Acupuncture was the first therapy with roots in Eastern philosophy to be accepted by orthodox medicine. Western doctors say it controls pain by releasing natural painkillers. But the philosophy behind it is based on a belief in more complex forces.*

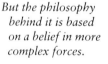

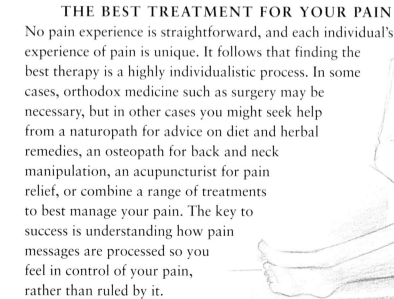

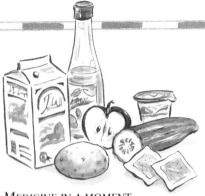

*MEDICINE IN A MOMENT*
*Most households contain a range of items which can relieve the discomfort or pain of everyday ailments. For example, sunburn can be relieved by cucumber, apple and potato, cold tea bags, milk or olive oil.*

*BEATING PAIN*
*If you let it, pain can ruin your life, forcing you to retreat into a world of isolation. With a positive mental attitude, however, you can dominate and control pain and continue to lead a full and active life.*

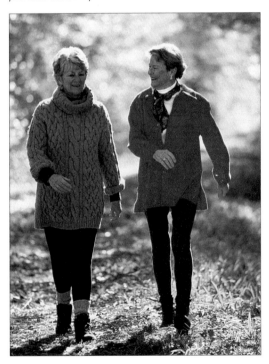

# MANAGING PAIN

The purpose of this book is to provide you with the ability to acknowledge and understand your pain and to enable you to make the right decisions on how to cope with it.

Chapter 1 explains the physiology of pain – how pain works, what causes it and why people experience the same pain differently. In Chapter 2 you will learn how to recognise pain as a warning system – what pain means, how serious it is, and when you should consult a doctor. In addition, there is a guide to combining conventional and natural treatments, along with a description of painkillers, both orthodox and natural.

Changing your lifestyle to prevent pain is covered in Chapter 3, with advice on balancing your diet, exercising, and adapting your habits to avoid pain. The array of traditional treatments now available to combat pain can cause some confusion; Chapter 4 describes how they can help to manage your pain more effectively.

Chapters 5 to 8 focus on different pains experienced in different parts of the body, giving the possible causes for each type of pain and the best approaches for them. In Chapter 5 you will find how to deal with headaches, earache, sore throats, toothache and some other less common ailments. Chapter 6 explains the causes of chest pain, ranging from a cough to angina, and abdominal pain. The pain from disorders of the reproductive and urinary systems is covered in Chapter 7. Advice is given for women's problems such as period pain, breast pain and pain related to uterine disorders; men will find information on problems that cause pain in the testes and penis. Chapter 8 describes ways to cope with back and neck pain, as well as painful joints, such as 'frozen shoulder' or 'tennis elbow'.

Chapter 9 aims to help those living with chronic pain and those who care for them, discussing the problems experienced by both and giving ideas on how to overcome them.

Finally, Chapter 10 offers first-aid advice for the pain caused by minor injuries, with alternative and conventional treatments for cuts, burns, bites and stings, sunburn and other minor ailments.

# Do you know how to manage your pain?

*Many people do not understand their pain and either use painkillers regularly or suffer in silence. But do you know what effect the painkillers are having? Do you know the latest advances in pain management? Do you know how to ease a headache or relieve back pain without using conventional painkillers? Few people realise the often simple steps they can take to avoid many types of pain.*

## Q WHEN WAS THE LAST TIME YOU TOOK A PAINKILLER?

If you are one of those people who pops a pill at the first sign of pain, then you could be damaging your health. While painkillers can be an effective remedy for short-term and non-recurring pain, their prolonged and excessive use can have unpleasant side effects (see Chapter 2). Added to this, by simply treating the pain itself, you are not dealing with its underlying cause. And prevention of pain is far better than the treatment of symptoms.

## Q ARE YOU UNSURE WHETHER TO CONSULT YOUR DOCTOR?

Many minor pains, if recurrent, can become an irritant in your life and you may be tempted to visit the doctor if you get no relief. However, pain can often arise from factors such as stress or diet that are within your power to control once you establish the trigger. For example, frequent migraines might be linked to something you eat, such as chocolate. Chapter 2 shows how keeping a pain diary allows you to build up a picture of when you feel the pain and what does or doesn't affect it. You may be able to take steps to correct the problem. If the pain seems to warrant medical attention, or if you experience any of the 'red flag' pain signals described in Chapter 2, then see your doctor. To prepare yourself for a consultation, complete the pain questionnaire and read the feature in Chapter 2 that explains the kind of questions your GP will ask you.

## Q DO YOU FEEL THAT MODERN MEDICINE HAS NO ANSWER TO YOUR PAIN?

Perhaps you have already visited doctors and specialists and been through a battery of tests without finding effective relief for your pain. If so, turn to Chapter 4. It is possible that one of the natural treatment methods may provide a potential answer to your problem. Bear in mind, however, that there are no miracle cures out there – it is simply a matter of finding what works best for you.

## Q DO YOU GET HEADACHES FREQUENTLY?

Headaches are the most common pain experienced in the United Kingdom with about 30 per cent of the population suffering them every year. The most common cause of headaches is stress and tension, usually as a result of today's hectic pace of life. Regular exercise is one of the most effective ways to dispel tension before it causes symptoms such as headaches. Relaxation techniques can also be invaluable in helping you to slow down. Chapter 5 gives details of other ways to prevent or relieve headaches.

## Q ARE YOU A BACKACHE SUFFERER?

Almost half the population of the United Kingdom suffer from backache at some time in their lives. Many people believe that backache is a fact of life and they despair of any real relief. But you don't have to give up – there are many measures you can take to alleviate this debilitating and often depressing condition. Chapter 8 describes how exercise can prevent and relieve backache, as well as giving sound advice on the many complementary medical treatments that can have an amazing impact on your back pain, such as massage, acupressure and osteopathy.

## Q ARE YOU LIVING WITH A CHRONIC PAIN SUFFERER?

It is estimated that 10 per cent or more of the populations of the United Kingdom and the United States suffer from chronic pain (medically defined as pain that occurs daily for more than three months). Carers of chronic pain sufferers know that it is hard to give the right amount of support without undermining the sufferer's independence. They also know that pain sufferers experience a range of emotions, including depression and fear, which can make the pain worse and further decrease a person's quality of life. The key to dealing with the emotional side of chronic pain is effective communication which promotes understanding – Chapter 9 offers pointers on how to achieve this. In addition, there is particular advice on caring for children and elderly people in pain.

# CHAPTER 1

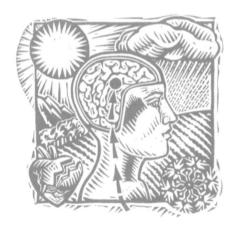

# WHAT IS PAIN?

*Pain is an unpleasant sensation that most of us do our best to avoid. It can vary in severity from mild discomfort to excruciating agony and can last for anything from just a few seconds to a lifetime. Although the primary function of pain is to protect the body from injury, there are other kinds of pain which are not so easy to define, such as the pain caused by disease.*

# THE PROCESS OF PAIN

*The process by which you experience pain is a complex one involving the brain and nerves. Understanding the mechanism, however, may help you to avoid or minimise your pain.*

**PAIN AS PROTECTION**
*Although pain is an unpleasant sensation, it actually functions to warn and protect the body from injury.*

An injury sends pain messages to the brain

**You feel the 'first' pain**

Your response is to protect yourself from the risk of further injury.

**You feel the 'second' pain**

Your response is to rest to allow the body to repair the damage.

Although pain is one of the most unpleasant of human experiences, it is, in fact, also one of the body's most important functions. You may not appreciate this when you experience a blinding headache, a throbbing toothache, or a cramping stomachache, but the pain is providing you with vital information about your current state of health or external risks to your health, and forcing you to rest so that healing can take place. A headache, for example, might be warning you that you are fatigued and stressed and need to rest; a toothache is probably informing you of damage to the tooth that needs to be attended to before more serious damage occurs; and the stomachache may be drawing your attention to poor dietary habits. Learning to understand and properly respond to your body's pain messages can help you to avoid many painful disorders.

## WHY YOU EXPERIENCE PAIN

When the body is injured, two types of pain are triggered. For example, if you twist your ankle, you immediately feel a sharp intense pain that grows worse in a matter of seconds and then rapidly begins to fade. This is known as the 'first' pain. Then another pain sensation, a deep, diffuse, sickening pain emerges and starts to spread slowly outside the affected region. This is known as the 'second' pain.

The first type of pain is a warning of possible injury, and the first response is to stop whatever is causing it. If this pain response didn't occur, then more serious injury could result. This type of pain also teaches you not to repeat certain actions, such as touching something hot. The dull sickening pain that follows makes you attend to the injury that has occurred. Without this second type of pain, there would be no motivation to protect the injured part from further harm,

or to rest and allow the body's own repair functions to take over and start mending the damage. Apart from making you rest – the oldest known cure – this kind of pain drives people to seek treatment.

However, there are other kinds of pain which do not seem to serve the purpose of warning the body. Pain may be triggered by causes which do not pose any threat at all to your well-being. For example, if you overexert yourself at the gym after a period of inactivity you will almost certainly have aching muscles the following morning. This is not because your body has experienced serious injury but because your muscles were not prepared for such a degree of exertion. Muscles prefer regular use and so exercising regularly will reduce the likelihood of experiencing this kind of pain.

In some cases the pain experienced can seem to be completely out of proportion to its cause. For example, passing a kidney stone can be extremely painful although the condition itself is not life-threatening.

The pain-warning system can also be triggered by such diseases as cancer and arthritis. This kind of pain appears to have no primary function, though it does encourage the sufferer to consult a doctor.

## HOW YOU FEEL PAIN

Pain messages are relayed from the injured area to the brain via the nervous system. The skin and deeper tissues of the body contain highly sophisticated nerve endings which sense changes outside and inside the body. These nerve endings can respond to external changes such as heat, cold or pressure, and to internal stimuli such as stretching and the release of chemicals from damaged cells. When these nerve endings are activated by direct stimuli, pain messages are sent to the brain. First they are relayed to an area in the spinal cord called

# NERVES AND THE BRAIN

The nervous system is a highly integrated mechanism that detects, analyses and responds to changes in conditions both inside and outside the body. The system is divided into two main parts: the central nervous system, which comprises the spinal cord and the brain; and the peripheral nervous system, which is made up of all the nerves that connect the brain and spinal cord to the rest of the body.

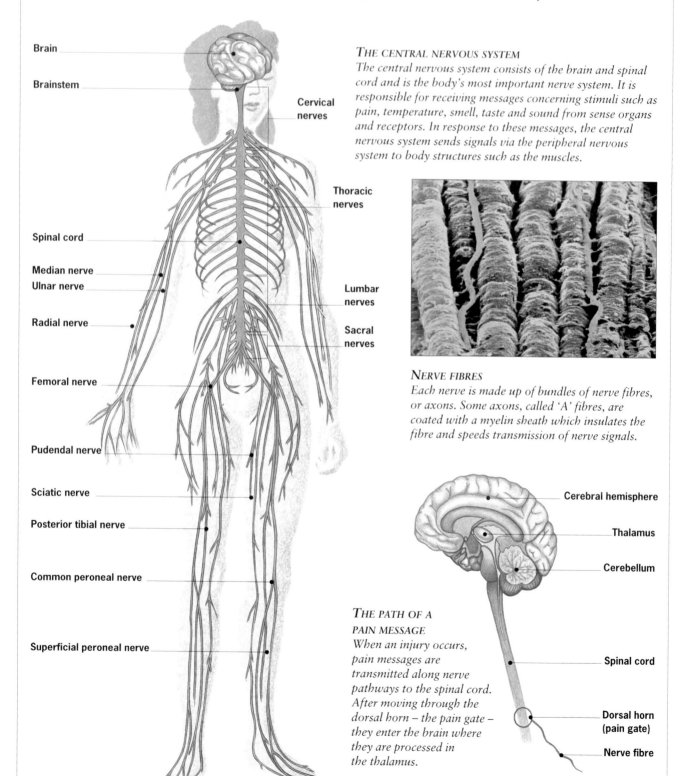

**Brain**

**Brainstem**

**Cervical nerves**

**Thoracic nerves**

**Spinal cord**

**Median nerve**

**Ulnar nerve**

**Lumbar nerves**

**Radial nerve**

**Sacral nerves**

**Femoral nerve**

**Pudendal nerve**

**Sciatic nerve**

**Posterior tibial nerve**

**Common peroneal nerve**

**Superficial peroneal nerve**

## THE CENTRAL NERVOUS SYSTEM
*The central nervous system consists of the brain and spinal cord and is the body's most important nerve system. It is responsible for receiving messages concerning stimuli such as pain, temperature, smell, taste and sound from sense organs and receptors. In response to these messages, the central nervous system sends signals via the peripheral nervous system to body structures such as the muscles.*

### NERVE FIBRES
*Each nerve is made up of bundles of nerve fibres, or axons. Some axons, called 'A' fibres, are coated with a myelin sheath which insulates the fibre and speeds transmission of nerve signals.*

**Cerebral hemisphere**

**Thalamus**

**Cerebellum**

**Spinal cord**

**Dorsal horn (pain gate)**

**Nerve fibre**

### THE PATH OF A PAIN MESSAGE
*When an injury occurs, pain messages are transmitted along nerve pathways to the spinal cord. After moving through the dorsal horn – the pain gate – they enter the brain where they are processed in the thalamus.*

## WHY AN INJURY FEELS TENDER

If you cut your finger you will usually find that the injured area feels inflamed and tender. Even a gentle touch to the area can be extremely painful. The inflammation of the area around the cut is caused by the release of chemicals such as prostaglandins from the damaged cells. These substances enlarge the blood vessels so that more blood plasma and cells can enter the tissues to start the healing process. The increased blood supply makes the area hot and as plasma collects in the tissue it starts to swell. The chemicals also cause exaggerated responses from the nerve endings in the injured area, so the cut feels tender even to the slightest touch. The pain serves to protect the area from further damage: because the injured part becomes more sensitive to pain, the body is forced to rest the damaged area to allow healing to take place.

*CROSS-SECTION OF A CUT*
*When you cut yourself, your body reacts immediately to repair the damage.*

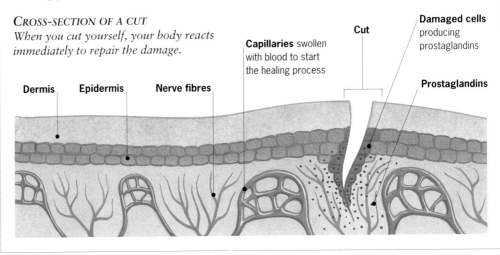

**Cut**

**Damaged cells** producing prostaglandins

**Capillaries** swollen with blood to start the healing process

**Prostaglandins**

**Dermis**   **Epidermis**   **Nerve fibres**

**'A' AND 'C' NERVE FIBRES**
*'A' fibres are surrounded by a thick insulating sheath which helps them to transmit pain messages more quickly. Messages transmitted on the 'C' fibres move more slowly. If the insulating sheath is destroyed, as occurs in multiple sclerosis, the nerve fibres cannot transmit impulses so numbness or weakness may result.*

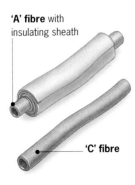

**'A' fibre** with insulating sheath

**'C' fibre**

the dorsal horn, where they are processed. From here the pain message travels up the spinal cord to the brain. Because all pain messages from the body pass through the dorsal horn before being transmitted to the brain, this part of the spinal cord is known as the 'pain gate'.

Once the pain message reaches the brain it is processed in an area called the thalamus, and pain is then experienced. Nerve impulses are then passed back from the brain to the muscles and internal organs to produce the response to pain in order to safeguard the individual.

The response to pain will be influenced by the properties of the tissue that is stimulated or damaged – for example, some parts of the body are more sensitive to stretching while others are more sensitive to extreme temperature or pressure. However, no matter what part of the body is stimulated or what the nature of the stimulation is, no pain can be felt without the brain – this is the reason why general anaesthesia is used during surgery. It works by neutralising the part of the brain that recognises pain.

### PRIORITISING PAIN MESSAGES

The brain is constantly bombarded with messages from different parts of the body giving information about changes occurring internally and externally. The thalamus deals directly with the most important sensory messages, such as those concerning pain, acting as a kind of filter. Other messages are transmitted from the thalamus to the outer layer of the brain, where the sensations are analysed. However, the body has its own system of making sure that important pain messages take priority to ensure the individual's safety.

This means that if the body faces injury from an external threat such as heat, priority will be given to the pain message so that the body can act immediately to deal with the potential threat. The body does this by transmitting urgent pain messages along nerve pathways, which conduct messages especially quickly. This produces the 'first' pain. These fast-conducting nerve pathways are known as 'A' fibres. Fibres that conduct pain messages more slowly are known as 'C' fibres. These produce the 'second' pain.

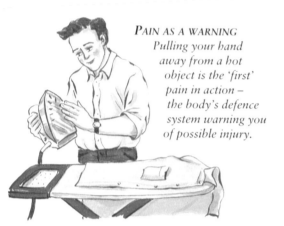

*PAIN AS A WARNING*
*Pulling your hand away from a hot object is the 'first' pain in action – the body's defence system warning you of possible injury.*

## The 'first' pain

The skin contains mostly fast-conducting 'A' fibres. This reflects the fact that the skin is the first line of defence against external threats to the body. For example, if a child places a hand too close to a candle flame the 'A' fibres in the skin will quickly send a pain warning message to the brain, even before injury has actually occurred. The brain processes the message and quickly reacts, instructing the muscles to pull the hand away from the flame to avoid injury.

## The 'second' pain

After the initial sharp warning signal, the duller, sickening pain message is passed along the slower-conducting 'C' fibres. 'C' fibres continue to transmit pain messages until the stimulus is removed and the tissue has recovered – and in some cases long after. The teeth and internal organs have mainly 'C' fibres, which explains why we are usually only aware of them when they are already damaged.

### PAIN AND THE BRAIN

Once the pain message has passed through the pain gate and on to the brain, it reaches the thalamus. This is where the various aspects of the pain message are analysed in order to determine appropriate action. However, the brain not only analyses the physical details of the pain message – such as where the pain is located, the form or type of pain, and any associated tenderness – it also takes into account other factors such as the emotional aspects of the pain experience, the unpleasantness of the pain, and its degree of severity.

Memory, too, is important in the overall processing of the pain message. The brain draws on earlier experiences of a similar pain, and on any stored knowledge about what such pain might mean, including pain experiences that have been reported by other people, in order to analyse the pain messages and arrive at an overall impression of the nature of the injury (see below).

### THE BODY'S OWN PAIN CONTROL SYSTEMS

If a child falls and bruises his or her knee, a mother's instinctive reaction is often to 'rub it better'. The mother may not realise it, but by simply rubbing the injured area she is causing the pain gate to close, thus preventing the transmission of any more pain messages to the brain. Rubbing the injured area stimulates other nerve fibres which feed into the dorsal horn with the pain messages. These impulses overload the pain gate so that eventually it becomes closed, causing the pain to diminish.

The body's own pain control system explains why the degree of pain felt is often at odds with the type of injury suffered. If, for example, you fall off your bicycle and scrape your hands and also break your wrist, initially you may only be aware of the pain from the cuts and grazes. This is because sensory overload has closed the pain gate, blocking access to 'C' fibre (or slow) pain impulses from damaged tissue around the bone which would indicate that

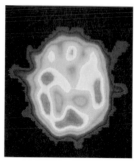

*PET SCAN*
*Pain perception can be studied using a technique called positron emission tomography (PET). This produces images which show the precise location of areas of brain activity. In the image above, the red areas indicate high activity and the blue areas show low activity. PET is being used to investigate the brain's reaction to pain and is greatly expanding our knowledge of the subject.*

## WHAT SHAPES PAIN PERCEPTION

Pain is felt entirely in the brain. But there are various external factors that contribute to any pain that we feel. The brain considers the psychological aspects of the injury as well as the actual physical damage when shaping the type of pain:

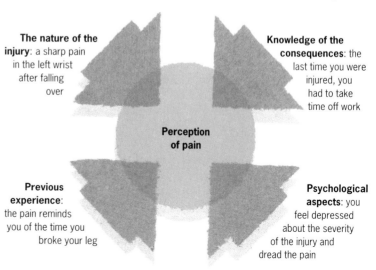

**The nature of the injury**: a sharp pain in the left wrist after falling over

**Knowledge of the consequences**: the last time you were injured, you had to take time off work

**Perception of pain**

**Previous experience**: the pain reminds you of the time you broke your leg

**Psychological aspects**: you feel depressed about the severity of the injury and dread the pain

## HOW TO UP YOUR ENDORPHINS

Research has shown that stimulation and pressure can encourage the release of endorphins, the body's natural painkiller. This may explain the benefit of oriental massage methods such as acupressure which focus on applying pressure to acupuncture points. You can help to increase the release of endorphins by:

▶ *Gently rubbing and moving the painful part.*

▶ *Taking exercise.*

▶ *Trying energy therapies such as acupuncture, acupressure and shiatsu.*

## ENDORPHIN PRODUCTION

As recently as 1973 scientists discovered that the body produces its own pain-relieving substances. Known as endorphins, these natural painkillers act in the brain, spinal cord and nerve endings at sites known as opiate receptors to relieve pain. In addition to their painkilling effect, endorphins are also believed to influence mood and regulate the body's response to stress.

**Injury** occurs and pain message is sent to brain → **Message is processed** → **Serotonin** is released → **Serotonin** stimulates endorphins → **Endorphins** block the transmission of pain messages to the brain

a more serious injury has taken place. By registering only that the skin has been cut, the brain is effectively prioritising pain messages: if the skin is damaged, there may still be an external threat that the body should move away from.

In the same way that the brain classifies pain messages according to importance, it also prioritises other messages quite unrelated to pain. For example, survival instincts are of paramount importance. If you are trapped in a burning building, your brain's priority is to help you to escape from the fire, rather than assess messages that your hand has been burnt.

Although this is an extreme example, pain management specialists are interested in the fact that the brain's ability to override pain has been observed during non-life-threatening situations such as sport. If a player is injured in a rugby match, it is often the case that he registers the pain of a serious injury only when the game is over. This is because the pain messages have been blocked as the brain perceives them as less important than the need to win the game.

If we can persuade the brain that winning a game of rugby is more important than acknowledging a torn ligament, we can also learn ways to persuade the brain that a constant message of arthritic pain is less important than, say, the desire to attend and enjoy a much-anticipated social event. Ways of achieving this are explored in Chapter 4.

### The body's own painkiller

The body produces its own painkillers in the form of chemicals known as endorphins. When pain messages reach the brain, the production of a chemical called serotonin is stimulated. Serotonin in turn helps to release endorphins which block the transmission of pain messages at specific sites, known as opiate receptors, located in the brain, nerves and spinal cord.

Recent research has established that a person's emotional state can influence the release of the endorphins. Stress and anxiety are known to inhibit the production of endorphins because the more depressed a pain sufferer is, the lower the level of serotonin produced, which in turn reduces the amount of endorphins released. The body's

## DEFENCE SYSTEMS

The brain is informed of changes in the environment by messages sent from highly sensitive nerve endings in the skin. These nerve endings, or nociceptors, have different sensitivities so some respond, for example, to extreme stimuli such as a cut, while others respond to changes in pressure.

*SENSORY OVERLOAD*
*The skin is particularly rich in nerve endings. Rubbing the injured skin after falling over may help to relieve pain by closing the pain gate.*

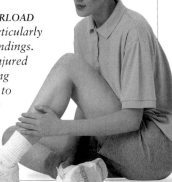

natural pain-coping mechanism is therefore diminished, because pain messages can be transmitted freely to the brain.

## TYPES OF PAIN

Although people can experience pain in many different ways, it is often helpful to consider two major categories of pain: acute and chronic.

### Acute pain

Everybody has had some experience of acute pain that can last a few days or in some cases a few weeks. This kind of pain is part of the body's response to injury or disease. Its primary purpose is to make us rest and allow healing to start. Physiological changes take place, such as increased pulse rate, raised blood pressure, sweating, a heightened awareness, and decreased response to other stimuli. Acute pain normally responds to painkillers, and the long-term effects of these are not a problem as they are usually only required for a short time.

### Chronic pain

Although acute pain has a purpose, chronic pain may continue for years with no benefit to the sufferer. Chronic pain may continue even after an initial injury has healed. It may also occur in response to a disease such as cancer or arthritis. Often the cause of chronic pain cannot be diagnosed.

Emotional and psychological factors play a significant role in the way you experience chronic pain. The brain analyses pain in terms of emotion as well as physiological experience, and emotions affect the body's release of endorphins. As a result, the more depressed and anxious you feel, the more intense the pain experience is likely to be.

It is also possible that chronic pain can become more severe due to 'conditioning'. The long-term experience of pain can lead to constant tensing of the muscles near the affected area. The nervous system may become conditioned to perceive pain whenever these muscle tension sensors are stimulated, so that any form of movement or exercise becomes painful.

The commonest cause of chronic pain is low back pain, followed by neck pain and arthritis. These pain problems tend not to respond well to pain-killing drugs.

### Referred pain

Pain from injury to the skin is usually felt precisely at the point of injury – it is said to be 'localised' – and often has a sharp, stinging quality. In contrast, pain from deep internal organs is hard to pinpoint and it is often difficult for people to describe exactly where they feel the pain. The symptoms are also quite different: the latter pain is deep and aching and often the sufferer feels nauseous and generally unwell.

## ACUTE PAIN AND CHRONIC PAIN

Acute pain is characterised by the rapid onset of symptoms, which can be extremely changeable, but last only a few days. In contrast, chronic pain describes pain that persists for a long time. The following physical and physiological differences between acute pain and chronic pain have been established.

| TYPE OF PAIN | PAIN EXPERIENCED | BODY RESPONSE | PHYSICAL CHANGES | TREATMENT |
|---|---|---|---|---|
| Acute pain | Often severe but normally of short duration (days) | Pain signals the body to rest so that damaged tissues can be repaired | The pulse rate becomes faster, the blood pressure rises, sweating increases, and there is a heightened sense of awareness and decreased response to other stimuli | Conventional painkillers work well, and are usually only required for a short time, enabling a resumption of activities |
| Chronic pain | Degree of pain often outweighs original cause. Link between source of pain and actual pain decreases as chronic pain continues over a long period (months/years) | Pain messages can still be generated long after initial stimuli have gone | If the nerve transmitting the pain messages is paired with muscle tensing pathways for a long time, the nervous system may become conditioned to perceiving pain whenever muscle tension sensors are stimulated | Herbal medicines used over a long period of time are often more effective than conventional painkillers; narcotics may demotivate. The sufferer's mental attitude and relationships can play a significant role in alleviating the pain |

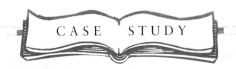

CASE STUDY

# Chronic Backache Sufferer

*Chronic backache is one of the commonest pain conditions. If back pain doesn't respond to the usual treatments given by a GP, fear of the consequences may lead to overprotection, which in turn can cause more pain. Strategies such as relaxation and gradually increasing activity can help the sufferer to cope with backache and lead a happier and more productive life.*

John is a successful 47-year-old businessman, with a wife, Ann, and three children. He developed backache following a football injury in his teens. His pain never troubled him until recently when it started to interfere with his activities. Work has become more stressful and he has had to stop playing squash as this makes his backache worse. He has become irritable and his relationship with Ann and his children has suffered. He is becoming increasingly worried about his inability to cope and his deteriorating relationship with his family. His doctor prescribed painkillers and rest, but these have had little effect. X-rays have revealed there is no surgically treatable cause for his backache.

## WHAT SHOULD JOHN DO?

John needs to consult a specialist at a pain management centre to develop a strategy to help him cope with his pain. His painkillers need to be reviewed, and he should think carefully about his lifestyle and emotional state. He needs to learn to pace his exercise, doing a little frequently rather than more strenuous exercise just once a week. He should practise relaxation techniques and study ways of managing his stress to help him to handle his workload, and to manage better with his pain. He needs to recognise that not getting along with his wife and children is adding to his stress and may be contributing to his condition. He should try to set aside more time to spend with them.

## Action Plan

**STRESS**
*Delegate work in the office and review responsibilities. Spend more time with the family, take up an interest and practise relaxation exercises on a regular basis.*

**FITNESS**
*Plan an exercise programme, set goals to increase physical activity. Targets could include swimming once a week with the family and helping Ann in the garden.*

**FAMILY**
*Make more use of the babysitter so that there is more time to spend alone with Ann. Plan more family outings.*

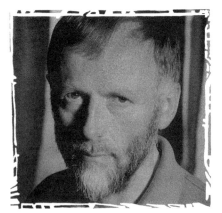

**FITNESS**
*Lack of exercise and inactivity causes a lack of confidence which in turn reduces tolerance to pain.*

**FAMILY**
*Chronic pain often causes difficulties within the family, sometimes leaving the sufferer isolated with the tendency to avoid activity for fear of increasing pain.*

**STRESS**
*Stress can cause increases in muscle tension that, when prolonged, can lead to more pain.*

## HOW THINGS TURNED OUT FOR JOHN

John reorganised work responsibilities and found he could leave the office earlier. He paced activities, didn't overexert himself, and spent more time with his family. As a result his confidence increased and in three months he was able to go for long walks, had taken up gardening and was becoming much more active. Although some of his pain persisted, his sleeping patterns improved and he was able to cope with it more effectively.

Pain from internal organs may be felt in other parts of the body, sometimes a great distance from the diseased or damaged area. This is known as referred pain. This occurs because a number of different parts of the body are supplied by the same nerve or group of nerves as the damaged tissues that are the source of pain. The brain can misinterpret or confuse the signals supplied from the same group of nerves. For example, pain caused by angina, where the heart muscle is starved of oxygen, is often referred to the arm: the heart and the arm are served by the same group of nerves.

## Describing pain

Within the broad definitions of acute and chronic pain, doctors further categorise pain into three distinctive types. The first type of pain, called somatic pain, occurs in the skin, muscles and bones. Generally it is constant and localised, and is characterised as aching, throbbing, or gnawing. Throbbing pain is often due to inflammation. Blood vessels dilate to increase the flow of blood to the area. With each pulse of blood a throb of pain occurs.

Pain from the inner organs of the body is called visceral pain. It is characteristically vague in distribution and quality, often described as deep, dull, aching, dragging, squeezing or pressure-like. When acute, it may be colicky. It can be due to distension of the smooth muscle walls of the intestine, rapid stretching of the enveloping sheath of organs such as the liver, or lack of blood supply and oxygen to tissue.

Neuropathic pain involves the nerves and can be further sub-divided into paraesthesia, dysaesthesia and allodynia. Pain may be due to the nerve being damaged as a result of injury or disease. It is often described as a burning sensation. Other symptoms commonly include tingling and numbness.

## DIFFERENT KINDS OF PAIN

Various parts of the body detect pain in different ways. The skin has a large number of pain receptors so injuries to the skin are felt acutely. The intestines, however, mainly contain receptors that detect when the tissues are being stretched. This means that distension resulting from excess gas, for example, is felt acutely, but a cut is not registered. Recognising the characteristics of pain can help to identify its cause.

| CHARACTERISTICS | TYPE | AREA | NAME | TYPICAL CAUSE |
|---|---|---|---|---|
| Aching, throbbing | Constant and localised | Skin, muscle, and bone | **Somatic** | Injuries to skin, muscle and bone such as cuts, bruises, burns and fractures; inflammation; vascular headaches |
| Deep, dull, dragging, squeezing, pressure-like; colicky | Vague in distribution and quality | Internal organs | **Visceral** | Distension of walls of intestine due to excess gas, wrong kind of food, lack of exercise or bowel inactivity after abdominal operation; lack of blood supply and oxygen and death of tissue. Colicky pain is caused by an overactive bowel brought on by too fierce or rapid contractions |
| Tingling with numbness, occasionally a burning sensation | Abnormal sensation without a stimulus | Nerve tissue | **Neuropathic** Paraesthesia (pins and needles) | Occurs when conduction of nerves from the body to the brain is partially blocked, for example, when the foot is in an awkward position for too long |
| Unpleasant, even intolerable sensation | Abnormal sensation | Nervous system | **Neuropathic** Dysaesthesia | Occurs with disease or injury to nervous system. |
| Hypersensitivity to stimulus such as touch | Pain is out of all proportion to light and touch stimulus. In extreme cases even the touch of clothing can cause extreme pain | Nervous system | **Neuropathic** Allodynia | Pain caused by prior damage of nerve endings, which makes the area oversensitive. Frequently accompanies damage to the nervous system, such as in the case of shingles |

# PERCEPTION OF PAIN

*The way the brain perceives pain is not only based on the actual physical sensation, it is also influenced by the individual's cultural background, personality and previous experience.*

Fast pain, which travels along the 'A' fibres, primarily has a warning function, signalling the body to take immediate action to protect itself from further injury. However, slow pain, which travels along the 'C' fibres, is processed in a more complex way: the brain draws on other types of information which influence its response to the pain message. These include memories of similar types of pain experienced before, how family members or friends may have coped with similar pains, and alarm about what the pain may lead to.

This means that the same kind of pain can be experienced in very different ways by different people according to factors such as their age, gender, culture and personality, as well as their previous experience of pain.

### INDIVIDUAL PAIN TOLERANCE

The term pain threshold refers to the level at which we experience pain when some kind of stimulus, such as pressure, is applied. Laboratory tests have shown that most people have a similar pain threshold. However, the level at which we label a pain as unbearable – known as our personal pain tolerance – varies significantly according to age, sex and cultural background.

Our perception of pain depends to a large degree on past experience and knowledge about what is likely to be painful. The more anxious or solicitous our parents are about any pain we may experience as children, the more we learn to fear pain. For example, if a parent is nervous and tense about how a child will cope with an injection and communicates this anxiety to the child, the child stores this information about injections, and comes to expect all injections to be painful. The brain's expectation of pain heightens the actual experience of pain.

In the same way, research has shown that an over-solicitous caregiver can reinforce the sufferer's perception of being in pain, which in turn heightens the brain's perception of actual pain.

The emotions play another important role in influencing our perception of pain. Being 'fussed over' by a carer may cause an emotional response in the patient, who learns subconsciously that a heightened sick role gains extra attention and care.

Negative emotions about pain can also heighten the sufferer's pain experience. Feelings of anxiety, fear and stress produce increased sensitivity to all external and internal stimuli, including pain. This aspect of pain perception is looked at in more detail on page 30.

## PAIN TOLERANCE AND THE INDIVIDUAL

The intensity of pain can vary from person to person, and also within the same person. Perception of pain varies according to the way you feel or the circumstances at the time. In addition, there are a variety of other factors that make the tolerance of pain unique to each individual.

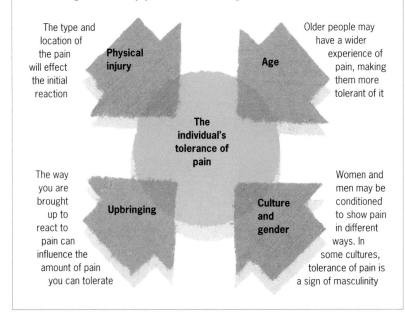

The type and location of the pain will effect the initial reaction

**Physical injury**

Older people may have a wider experience of pain, making them more tolerant of it

**Age**

**The individual's tolerance of pain**

The way you are brought up to react to pain can influence the amount of pain you can tolerate

**Upbringing**

**Culture and gender**

Women and men may be conditioned to show pain in different ways. In some cultures, tolerance of pain is a sign of masculinity

## Cultural differences in feeling and dealing with pain

People from different cultural backgrounds have been shown to react differently to the experience of pain, even when the injury or illness causing the pain is the same. Although the pain threshold is similar, the outward expression of pain may differ enormously. In some cultures, people express their feelings openly and visible expressions of pain and discomfort are positively encouraged. In other cultures, people are conditioned to hide or mask their feelings and may not be encouraged to express pain openly. For example, by tradition Japanese women are not expected to vocalise their pain during childbirth.

Richard Sternbach, a psychologist specialising in pain in California, studied the pain tolerance levels among a group of American women from various ethnic backgrounds in order to determine the influence of their cultural background on experimental pain. His research revealed that women of Italian descent, who openly voiced their suffering, tolerated less pain than women of British or Jewish origin.

An understanding of the ways in which your cultural background can affect your pain perception and pain tolerance may help you to gain control over your own reaction to pain and devise strategies to control the amount of pain you feel.

## Gender differences in feeling and dealing with pain

Gender and age influence how people react to pain. In many cultures, males are encouraged to be more stoical and reserved. If they have a physical problem that is causing pain they are not encouraged to complain about it. Any outward display of pain or suffering may be taken as a sign of weakness or insecurity. In contrast, women are more able to discuss their emotions openly and as a result of this may display pain and suffering to a greater degree.

Some cultures go so far as to regard the ability to withstand pain without showing any reaction as a sign of great manliness, and so adolescent boys are encouraged to demonstrate their high pain tolerance. The same ability in a young woman, however, is seen as unfeminine and so discouraged.

Pain clinics (see page 69) usually have a slightly higher proportion of women attendees than men. This may be due in part to the fact that women are more likely to seek

### Munchausen's syndrome

In extreme cases, enjoyment of the sick role can lead to Munchausen's syndrome, a psychological disorder where the sufferer complains of pain that is pretended or self-induced. In some cases sufferers may actually experience pain, so strong is the conditioning of their subconscious mind. Physical symptoms may include fever, skin rashes, dizziness, and pain in the abdomen. Patients are usually well versed in medical matters and often bear the scars of previous treatments or investigations. In Munchausen's syndrome by proxy, parents insist that their children are suffering from painful medical conditions.

---

## CULTURAL DIFFERENCES IN PAIN PERCEPTION

Although the intensity of pain may be the same, how the pain is expressed and the way we cope varies according to our background. In some cultures internalising emotions is encouraged but in others an extravagant display of feelings may be standard. The different film styles of northern and southern Europe show how culture can condition the expression of emotions and pain.

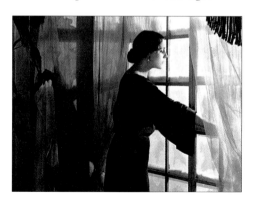

**NORTHERN REPRESSION**
*The bleak landscapes, languid movements and solemn expressions typical of films made in northern Europe are symbolic of the internalised emotions of their characters.*

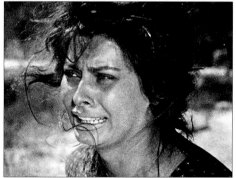

**SOUTHERN EXPRESSION**
*Dramatic or passionate gestures and displays of high emotion are common features in films of southern Europe or Latin America, reflecting the expressive nature of the culture.*

## Origins

The influence of environment, experience and knowledge on our perception of pain has been the subject of many studies this century. Dr Henry K. Beecher, who later became the first Professor of Anaesthetics at Harvard University, was involved with treating soldiers during the Second World War. He observed that soldiers wounded in battle were much less likely to ask for or need morphine than civilians who had received similar injuries. The difference lay in the emotional response: whereas the soldier felt relief at escaping from the battlefield alive, the civilian saw the injury as a depressing and calamitous event. As a result Beecher came to the conclusion that 'there is no simple direct relationship between the wound per se and the pain experienced'. His theory explains why a person can feel the same pain differently according to the environment and current mental and emotional state. For example, a child will laugh if smacked in play but cry if the same slap is given as a punishment.

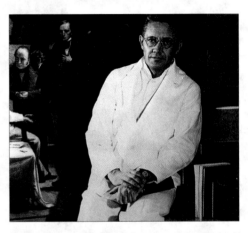

DR HENRY K. BEECHER (1904–76)
Dr Beecher was one of the foremost researchers into the perception of pain.

**Does a foetus feel pain?**
From the 20th week of pregnancy a foetus begins to show response to painful stimuli. Initially, these responses are more like primitive reflexes, but as the nervous system matures, the responses become more specific to the area of stimulation. Thus it can be assumed that a foetus feels pain in the same way that any animal showing such a response to a painful stimulus would be considered to be experiencing pain.

help for a pain problem than men. Studies have shown that women are more likely to report chronic pains that are more severe and last for a longer period. Also, according to experiments women generally report pains in a wider range of areas than men.

Recent research suggests that the gender difference in pain perception may actually have a specifically biological basis, as well as a cultural one. In experiments carried out on a group of men and women who had just had their wisdom teeth removed, medical researchers in California discovered that opiate painkillers had a longer-lasting effect on the women than on the men. This research could have major implications for the way that men and women are treated for pain in the future.

### Age differences in feeling pain
Age, too, has a bearing on how pain may be perceived. The older a person is, the more likely he or she is to have experienced a wide range of acute and chronic pain conditions. As a result, the person is more likely to have developed a higher degree of tolerance and can also draw on past experience in order to recognise the pain and come to terms with it and manage it.

### How children communicate pain
Children are not as articulate in describing their pain as adults. They have less knowledge and experience to draw on to determine what kind of pain they are feeling. Thus a pain anywhere may be described as a 'tummy-ache', or nausea may be described as a 'sore throat'. Pain may also be communicated through other means such as temper tantrums, crying, sulking and resorting to behaviours such as bedwetting. It may not be clear if a child is experiencing pain, generalised distress, or simply trying to get attention. For example, a child experiencing problems at school may develop 'pains' in order to stay at home.

Children may find it easier to communicate their pain and its location through drawings. These can help the doctor to diagnose the problem more accurately.

Children may mimic their parents' or older siblings' reaction to pain. Similarly, they may develop the same fear of pain shown by other family members. In a child this is accentuated by a lack of emotional maturity and inability to rationalise fears. Parents should always be aware of their reactions to both their own pain and that of their children.

# THE CAUSES OF PAIN

*We usually think of pain as being caused by a specific injury or disease. However, pain can arise from other causes which an individual can learn to control or avoid.*

Physical pain is frequently caused by injury to the body. Chemicals such as prostaglandins are released after injury to help the healing process get underway. Paradoxically, these chemicals intensify the pain because they stimulate the nerve endings to transmit pain messages to the brain. These messages have a protective function as they induce the body to rest the injured area to allow the damaged tissues to be repaired.

Localised physical pain may also be experienced as a direct result of tissue damage caused by disease. For example, a tumour pressing on or disturbing a nerve can cause pain. However, illness and disease can also cause a more generalised pain response – even if there is no actual tissue damage. Generalised myalgia, or painful aching of the muscles, is commonly experienced during a bout of influenza and warns the body of the need to rest.

Pain is almost inevitable after surgery. It may be minimised, however, by the skill of the surgeon and the anaesthetist, and by the knowledge that the pain is only temporary while healing occurs.

### PAIN DURING EXERCISE

Although exercise is vital for keeping the muscles active and promoting general good health, pain can arise both during and after exercise. If you do brisk exercise after a long period of inactivity, your muscles will probably be tender and actually feel swollen several hours later. This type of pain is due to mechanical damage of the muscles. You can avoid this by warming up your muscles before exercise, and by building up your exercise programme gradually.

If you find that chest pain comes on during exercise and rapidly increases until the activity has stopped, you may be suffering from narrowing of the arteries which is causing a limited blood supply to reach the heart. Narrowing of the arteries can be caused by high blood pressure or high

## EXERCISE PAIN AS A WARNING

To avoid pain when exercising, start off by keeping well within your capabilities and steadily build up over a number of sessions as your fitness levels improve. Stop exercising at once and see your doctor if you experience any of the following symptoms:

▶ *A fast pumping heart beat that persists for five minutes after exercise has stopped.*

▶ *Pain in the arm, neck or chest.*

▶ *Severe joint pain.*

▶ *Severe breathlessness.*

▶ *Feeling faint.*

## WARMING UP

Warming up exercises are an essential part of any exercise routine. Gentle, rhythmic movements such as stretching prepare the heart, lungs and muscles for more strenuous work to come. Warming up also helps to lubricate the joints so they can work more efficiently when you start your exercise programme. If you don't warm up sufficiently, you may suffer dizziness, muscle cramps and chest pains. Cooling down is just as important – gentle movements after an exercise session help the blood flow to return to normal. To warm up and cool down, try the illustrated exercise.

*THE SWAN*
*Bend the knees with feet wide apart. Put your right hand on the hip, left above the head and lean to the right. Repeat in in both directions several times.*

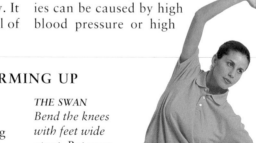

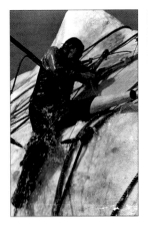

***CAPTAIN AHAB AND PHANTOM PAIN***
*One of the most famous literary figures to suffer phantom pain was Captain Ahab in Herman Melville's epic novel* Moby Dick *(1851). The legendary whaler lost a leg in a terrifying accident but continued to feel frequent bouts of agonising pain in the limb that had been removed. The picture above shows Gregory Peck as Captain Ahab in the 1956 film version of the story.*

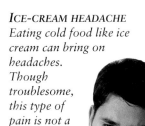

***ICE-CREAM HEADACHE***
*Eating cold food like ice cream can bring on headaches. Though troublesome, this type of pain is not a cause for serious concern.*

# PHANTOM PAIN

People who have lost a limb often feel as if the limb is still there, because the nerve pathways serving that part of the body are still transmitting messages to the brain. They may also experience pain in the part of the body that has been removed, which relates to pain in that area prior to amputation. The pain is no less real than if the limb was still in place. This condition is known as phantom pain and is usually described as crushing, cramping or burning. The pain may persist as long as the nerve pathways continue to transmit pain messages. Phantom pain usually dissipates in time. In some cases, however, the pain is severe and does not decrease. Transcutaneous electrical nerve stimulation (TENS) has been shown to relieve phantom pain in many cases (see page 83).

blood cholesterol levels, smoking, diabetes and obesity. If you fit into any of these categories, consult your doctor before starting an exercise programme.

## DYSFUNCTION OF PAIN NETWORK

Damage to nerves can lead to a malfunctioning of the pain network. Pain symptoms can occur when a nerve or nerve pathway is damaged. Even minor injuries can lead to extensive, persistent pain problems if the nerve pathway relevant to the affected area is damaged. In such cases the nerve pathway becomes hyper-excitable, sending erratic pain messages to the brain for no apparent reason. Similar sensations are frequently experienced by people who have lost a limb (see above).

## THE EFFECTS OF COLD

In extreme cold weather, you may find that your fingers and toes begin to ache. This is because in subzero temperatures, the arteries supplying the fingers and toes can go into spasm, restricting blood flow and releasing chemicals which send warning pain messages to the brain. Even if you warm the affected area, the pain will persist until all the chemicals released in connection with the muscle spasm have been cleared. In some cases, cold can cause minor, but often painful complaints such as chilblains and chapped skin. Chilblains are caused by too rapid rewarming of the skin after it has been exposed to extremely cold conditions. Chapped skin occurs most frequently in cold weather when oil-secreting glands produce less oil to lubricate the skin. In severe cases persistent lack of blood flow due to cold leads to tissue damage, as in frostbite, or tissue death, as in gangrene.

## PAIN IN MENTAL ILLNESS

Sometimes people suffer such severe psychological trauma that it is actually experienced as physical pain. There may be several reasons for this response. Physical pain rather than a psychological problem is often easier for a patient's family to accept. Or sometimes the role of the invalid is seen as offering greater benefits, such as sympathy or a chance to avoid responsibilities. In extreme cases, the body copes with painful emotions by converting them into physical pain. For example, a man who has caused injury to another with his right arm might be so traumatised that he too will start to feel pain in his right arm. Although the pain originates in the mind it feels completely genuine to the sufferer. Known as conversion disorder, this problem is usually resolved by coming to terms with the underlying psychological problem.

Some people develop delusions that their body has altered in some way, for example, that an arm is being eaten away or disfigured. Pain may accompany such delusions, which are common in schizophrenics.

## SELF-MUTILATION

Self-mutilation, the act of deliberately cutting or otherwise injuring yourself, often involves pain. It is common among people suffering with depression, schizophrenia, bulimia nervosa or feelings of hostility. The need to relieve tension, the influence of alcohol or other substances, aggressive impulses or a desire for attention are some of the possible reasons for self-mutilation.

# SELF-INFLICTED PAIN

Cultural factors are known to affect the way pain is perceived. This is evident in traditional customs and sacred rites where pain plays a part, such as tattooing, body-piercing, and mutilation for religious reasons. For example, the ceremony of hook-swinging, practised in parts of India, involves suspending a male member of the community from hooks that have been embedded in his back. The man seems to suffer no pain during the ceremony but rather appears to be in a state of exaltation.

In Western culture, body-piercing and tattooing may be a way of promoting self-identity, or group affinity. Some people who have undergone body-piercing report a pleasant sensation at the time of piercing, described as a 'rush' or 'high', that can last several hours. This may be due to the release of endorphins, the body's own painkiller.

The states of pleasure and pain and the thin line dividing them have been much discussed by philosophers since the days of Plato. Ecstasy is commonly understood to be a state of intense delight, although, as in 'the agony and the ecstasy' of Christ, it also refers to the overwhelming state of any emotion such as fear or pain. This overwhelming state is somewhat similar to a trance. The suffering may be endured as a means of obtaining the heightened state.

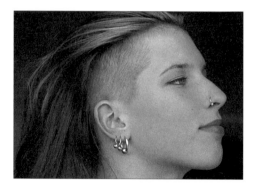

*BODY PIERCING*
*Piercing the body with a variety of objects is a common phenomenon throughout the world. In some cultures this kind of piercing may be linked to initiation rites, indicating that a male or female has reached a certain phase in maturity. In the West, ear piercing became fashionable in the 1960s and today piercing other parts of the body, such as the nose or the navel, is becoming increasingly common.*

*FIREWALKING*
*Rituals involving fire, such as walking over hot coals, as shown here in Sri Lanka, are found all over the world. Many cultures believe that firewalking is a test of faith and firewalkers claim that they are aided by strength of belief. Scientists believe that a crucial factor in successful firewalking is the amount of time that the foot is in contact with the coals. However, there is no doubt that willpower also plays an important part in distracting the mind and blocking the pain.*

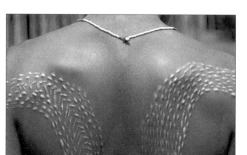

*RITUAL SCARRING*
*The practice of producing raised scars on the human body in decorative patterns is particularly common in parts of Africa and Melanesia and among Australian aborigines. The scarring may indicate an individual's status or tribal allegiance or it may be done purely for cosmetic reasons. The patterns are produced by cutting with a knife or sometimes by burning. In some cases objects, such as protective charms, may be placed under the skin.*

## Sadomasochism
Sadomasochism is an abnormal condition in which sexual pleasure derives from the infliction (sadism) and receipt (masochism) of pain. The term can refer to the combination of both sadism and masochism in one person, or a couple may indulge in sadomasochistic practices whereby one partner has heightened sexual arousal from inflicting pain and the other derives pleasure from receiving it.

# EMOTIONAL PAIN

*Emotional pain is experienced completely within the brain, but painful physical symptoms often follow because of the close link between the brain and the physical functioning of the body.*

**Mind over body**
According to statistics, there is a significant fall in the number of deaths of patients suffering a terminal illness before important events such as birthdays and festivals. The fact that people are able to delay death in order to be present at a celebration illustrates the power of mind over body. This forms the basis of visualisation therapy: the mind can be trained to exercise more control over the body.

Emotional pain can have many causes, for example grief over the loss of a loved one, or feelings of rejection after divorce, or shock at being 'unwanted' following redundancy. Such emotional trauma can lead to depression and anxiety and, in extreme cases, to physical pain as the areas of the brain that process emotional pain and suffering are the same as those that deal with physical pain.

For example, after being rejected by a partner, amongst the complicated mixture of emotions – anger, hurt, betrayal – is a feeling of threat and insecurity. Once a threat message has been perceived by the brain a typical stress 'fight or flight' response is activated: muscles tense, the heart rate increases and soon the individual feels tense as well as hurt and unhappy. After the initial shock fades, many people pass through phases of profound sadness, anger, guilt, depression, helplessness, confusion, and erratic or impulsive behaviour. Physical symptoms are often similar to those experienced under stress: appetite loss and insomnia are both common.

### HOW EMOTIONS AFFECT PAIN
Your emotional state can strongly influence the sensation of pain. According to your feelings and character, your response to an initial pain message can either intensify and prolong the pain experience or it may reduce the amount of pain perceived.

### Anxiety and pain
Anxiety about the pain you are feeling or anticipate feeling has been shown to intensify the perception of pain. When a group of medical students were told they were

## THE VICIOUS CYCLE OF PAIN

Your perception of pain is closely linked to your thoughts and behaviour. Emotions such as anxiety can actually heighten the perception of pain leading to further stress and negative emotions, which in turn cause further pain.

**Feeling anxious** about the consequences of your condition can actually make you more sensitive and increase your pain

**Fear and uncertainty** about the nature of your condition can make pain receptors more sensitive, increasing the perception of pain

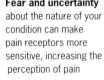

**Depression** caused by a long standing condition can heighten your pain by inhibiting the production of endorphins

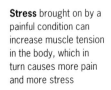

**Stress** brought on by a painful condition can increase muscle tension in the body, which in turn causes more pain and more stress

## THE LANGUAGE OF EMOTIONAL PAIN

The extent to which physical manifestations of emotional pain affect us is reflected in the language we use to describe painful emotional states. Statements such as 'I felt as though my heart would break' indicate how emotional pain can be transferred to a physical experience. Many people describe their initial reaction to the death of a partner or friend as a feeling of numbness. This feeling has been described as the 'heart's analgesic' and may be the brain's way of playing for time before admitting the loss of a loved one and having to come to terms with the intense emotional pain associated with it.

going to be subjected to high levels of pain when asked to hold hot metal rods, the students grimaced and dropped the rods even though they were not hot at all.

When you feel anxious, you tend to feel much more sensitive to external and internal stimuli – for example, noises may seem louder and lights brighter. This can heighten your perception of pain and make it feel worse. Relaxation and being well informed about any pain you may be about to feel can help to dispel anxiety and so reduce the amount of pain you experience.

Anxiety about something other than your own problems, however, can serve to distract you from pain. It is not uncommon for people with chronic backache to find their experience of pain diminishes if a close family member falls seriously ill.

### Depression and pain

Depression can make pain feel worse, particularly if it is long-standing. This is partly because depression can reduce the body's ability to produce endorphins.

In severe cases of depression people may become completely preoccupied with their physical problems. They may come to believe that part of their body is damaged or altered in some way and causing severe pain. In such cases the pain is actually caused by the underlying depression.

### Fear and pain

If you don't know the cause of a pain, the fear and uncertainty may increase the pain itself. As with anxiety, fear heightens the body's receptiveness to stimulation making pain receptors more sensitive. Sometimes people avoid doing exercise for fear that strenuous activity might cause an injury, even though exercise might be beneficial. People recovering from a heart attack, for example, are often advised to exercise. They might notice that their heart rate goes up following exercise and, although this is quite a normal response, they may interpret the raised heart rate as signalling the onset of another heart attack. The resulting panic causes the heart rate to rise even more and they may even develop pain symptoms.

### Stress and pain

Stress can increase the experience of pain and make it more difficult to cope. When you find yourself in a stressful situation, your body responds by increasing the production of certain hormones such as adrenaline. These hormones cause a variety of changes in the body, including raising the blood pressure and heart rate. When stress is experienced over a prolonged period, the body's reaction is to tense the muscles. Muscles in a state of sustained tension in the neck, shoulders and head can cause pain, which then causes more stress and more tension, thus increasing the pain. Tightening of the muscles in the face, scalp and neck can cause tension headaches, which can last anything from hours to weeks.

Making a conscious effort to relax and reduce your stress levels is often recommended as a way of decreasing the risk of pain from stress-related problems. There are various relaxation therapies (see pages 91 and 92) you can try that can help to prevent some of the first signs of stress such as shallow breathing, lack of concentration and disturbed sleep, which can all heighten your perception of pain.

### DEALING WITH EMOTIONAL PAIN

Most counsellors and therapists agree that profound emotional pain is best confronted head on:

▶ *Don't hide or repress your feelings, otherwise they may re-emerge in physical stress-related disorders such as eczema and tension headaches.*

▶ *Discuss your emotions openly with a friend or counsellor.*

▶ *Consciously call a halt to negative feelings – these can generate chemical reactions in the brain leading to a cycle of depression.*

▶ *Try to focus on the positive aspects of your life.*

▶ *Pinch yourself, literally, to direct your brain away from negative thoughts.*

▶ *Try visualising yourself in a relaxing scene such as on holiday or in a pleasant environment.*

# COPING WITH FEAR

*Fear of the unknown, feelings of uncertainty and lack of understanding can all make pain feel worse. In some cases fear of pain can be worse than the actual pain itself.*

The way you experience pain is greatly influenced by your upbringing, experiences, education and culture. If you feel frightened by the pain you are suffering or the treatments that you are about to undergo, the fear may prevent you from thinking and behaving rationally. However, perhaps most significantly, fear and anxiety will actually heighten your pain experience (see page 30). Although changing deeply entrenched attitudes to pain is not easy, learning to cope with and minimise fear is one of the most important pain management strategies you can acquire.

## WHY WE DEVELOP FEAR OF PAIN

Fear of pain most often develops in childhood when we are less able to analyse experience in a rational manner. While an adult may understand the need for a certain amount of pain to be experienced in order to benefit in the long term, a child may find it difficult to appreciate the value of pain when set against the fear it causes. One bad experience in childhood such as a very painful injection at the dentist can cause long-standing fears which continue into adulthood. Anxiety exaggerates the initial fear, and may lead to avoidance which in turn exacerbates the fear and anxiety.

Having an operation or other medical treatments and tests may produce fear not only of the pain but of what may be done to the individual, and in what state the individual will be left even after recovery. Fear of ongoing treatment, fear of recurrence of the problem, and fear of what will happen if treatment is unsuccessful, all contribute to general anxiety about pain.

The role that fear plays in increasing pain is perhaps most clearly seen with victims of torture. Victims report that the anticipation of pain is worse than the actual infliction of pain. The work of Amnesty International has highlighted the disintegration of the personality that results from prevention of sleep, the expectation that the pain will be worse each time it is inflicted, and the fear that the torture will become more severe as the process continues.

## HOW TO AVOID FEAR

The experience of torture victims highlights one of the most important aspects of pain management: when people feel they have some control over the amount of pain they experience, they are able to tolerate higher levels of pain. When others are responsible for inflicting the pain, however, the level of pain tolerated drops dramatically, primarily due to anxiety. This phenomenon has also been proven in scientifically controlled experiments. The first step in coping with fear of pain must therefore be to become as informed as possible about every aspect of your condition and treatment: what it

*continued on page 36*

## PREPARING A CHILD FOR AN OPERATION

The key to preparing a child for a painful operation is communication. Open talking and explanations of what is going to happen are likely to make young patients feel relaxed and more secure. If your child is young, you can explain medical procedures using familiar toys. Talking through a puppet and drawing pictures may also encourage children to talk and express their feelings.

*GIVING SUPPORT*
*Using a familiar toy to explain procedures can help to allay a child's fears.*

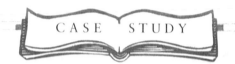

# Fear of the Dentist

*A single unpleasant experience during dental treatment as a child can lead to a fear that stays with you for life. Your anxiety may force you to avoid all dental appointments, but this will only make the fear worse and may have serious consequences for your teeth. By gradually facing up to the feared situation, and using relaxation and coping techniques, you can learn to overcome your fear.*

Paula is 14 years old and living with her parents and younger brother. She is doing well at school, and enjoys sport. She developed a fear of dentists as a young child after experiencing a painful tooth extraction. As she has got older the fear has become worse. Paula's mother has been trying to get her to go to the dentist but she is frightened herself and this has prevented her from forcing her daughter to go. Paula developed a severe toothache recently and after much persuasion went to see her dentist. She managed to sit in the waiting room but when she was about to be examined by the dentist, panicked and rushed out in tears. Although the toothache persisted she could not face having treatment.

## WHAT SHOULD PAULA DO?

Paula needs to feel more in control of the situation. Together with her parents she should discuss a strategy for coping with a visit to the dentist. Paula should visit the surgery before making an appointment so she can familiarise herself with the waiting area and the examination room without having the anxiety of treatment. She should also discuss with the dentist exactly what the treatment involves and how long it will take. To feel further in control, Paula should agree on some kind of hand signal with the dentist, so that if she does feel pain she can make a sign for the dentist to stop. Paula also needs to learn and practise visualisation and breathing techniques to help her to relax.

## Action Plan

**STRESS**
*Practise breathing and relaxation techniques on a regular basis. Visualise scenes which will help to distract the mind from pain.*

**FAMILY**
*Family members should not show anxiety which might influence behaviour. Watch other people successfully undergoing treatment to help to develop ways of coping.*

**HEALTH**
*Find out about the treatment, how long the procedure will last, and what the effects will be. Find out about the consequences of not undergoing the treatment.*

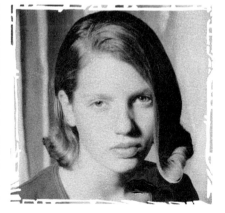

**FAMILY**
*The reaction of family members can influence the response to pain and feared events.*

**HEALTH**
*A poor understanding of a feared event will increase anxiety levels, which in turn can increase the amount of pain you feel.*

**STRESS**
*Stress causes heightened anxiety and tension which can result in muscle spasm.*

## HOW THINGS TURNED OUT FOR PAULA

Paula practised relaxation exercises. Taking deep breaths while visualising lying on a secluded beach helped her to relax. She discussed her treatment step-by-step with her dentist, and arranged a hand signalling procedure. She successfully underwent a dental examination and the anxiety slowly decreased over subsequent sessions. Although she never had to use the hand signal, she felt more in control knowing it was available.

*Preparing yourself for*

# A Painful Event

*There are strategies you can adopt to help you to cope as you approach a potentially painful event. They will lessen the fear and anxiety and help you to feel more in control. In turn, this should diminish the pain and aid recovery.*

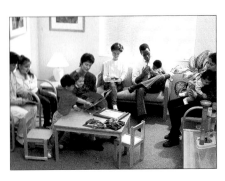

**FEELING AT HOME**
*Familiarising yourself with the surgery and waiting room and assuring yourself that there are others in the same situation as yourself can help to reduce your fears.*

There are several things you can do to prepare yourself for a potentially stressful treatment or consultation at a clinic or hospital.

Make sure you know exactly what the treatment will involve by discussing what will happen with your doctor. If possible, it may help to visit the hospital or surgery before treatment to help you to get used to the environment. Many people find it comforting to have a friend or relative present at the consultation but in some cases this has been shown to heighten the perception of pain (see page 19).

### THE NIGHT BEFORE

Being relaxed and well organised can help you to prepare for a stress-free visit to the doctor. It is important to start your preparations the night before. Write down a short description of your condition to date, making it as clear and accurate as possible. If you've been noting down your pain symptoms in a diary (see page 44), it would be helpful to bring that along, too. Think rationally about your condition and write down any questions that you would like to ask as they may easily slip your mind during the consultation. Don't forget to pack a notebook and pencil in your bag, too, to note down any information about your treatment or dosages of medications.

If you are feeling anxious, practise relaxation and breathing exercises. For example, visualising yourself in the feared situation and then imagining a successful outcome can help you to gain confidence and overcome your fears of the impending treatment. To decrease your anxiety levels relax in a hot bath with favourite music and perfumed candles. It's also a good idea to avoid caffeine as this can increase anxiety and pain.

Finally, when your bag is packed, have a cup of hot milk, or a herbal tea such as camomile or rosehip, and go to bed early. A good night's sleep the night before the treatment can make all the difference for a trouble-free visit to the doctor.

### WAKING UP

When you wake up on the morning of your treatment, make sure your first thoughts are positive.

▶ *Breathe deeply, relax and then flex your muscles.*

▶ *Make a mental list of the things that you enjoy about life and the attributes that others value in you.*

▶ *Think about the good things that happened to you the previous day and imagine that tomorrow you can add the treatment to the list.*

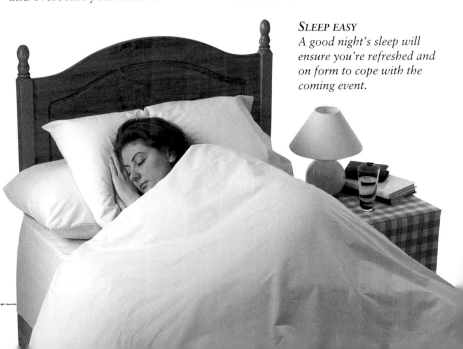

**SLEEP EASY**
*A good night's sleep will ensure you're refreshed and on form to cope with the coming event.*

One way of reducing fear of pain is to be as informed as possible about the treatment options available to you. Talk to your caregivers and don't be afraid to discuss your health and ask probing questions about surgery and medication. The following questions cover the main points, but there may be other issues you want to raise:

## BE INFORMED

▶ *Do I understand the treatment step-by-step?*

▶ *How long will the treatment last?*

▶ *How long will the short-term effects last?*

▶ *What are the effects and outcome expectations of the treatment?*

▶ *Is there a chance that more pain might be caused?*

▶ *Are there any other treatment options available such as pain clinics, osteopaths, physiotherapists, chiropractors, alternative healers?*

▶ *Are there any risks associated with the treatment?*

▶ *Will I be allowed to control the amount of painkilling medications that are prescribed?*

## WHILE YOU'RE THERE

Make sure you enter the doctor's surgery believing that it will turn out to be a successful visit. If you make yourself believe that the outcome will be negative, very often the visit will turn out to be so. In the same way, imagining positive scenarios can help to engender a positive outcome. While you're waiting to see the doctor, you can help to distract your mind by reading a magazine or chatting to a fellow patient.

Practising a visualisation exercise (see page 141) can also help you to relax. Imagining a pleasant scene will distract you from any pain and help you to think more positively about the treatment you are about to undergo. Sit as comfortably as possible keeping your head, neck and body straight but relaxed. Keep your eyes closed or focus on some neutral site and try to imagine the pain as being far away and not part of you. In this way it may be possible to develop a feeling of detachment from the pain. You can choose any visual image that you find has a calming influence.

If you have difficulty in choosing a suitable image, it may help to bring along an illustrated book. Try looking at a picture for three or four minutes, then close the book and try to remember exactly what was going on in the picture. How many people were there? What were they doing? What colours were used? How would you have painted the picture if

you had been the artist? Alternatively take a novel with you and try to imagine how you would make a film of the story you're reading. Children respond particularly well to visualisation techniques because they usually have very vivid imaginations.

Breathing exercises (see page 142) may also be effective at calming you while you're waiting. Breathe in and imagine the breath travelling through your entire body down to the tips of

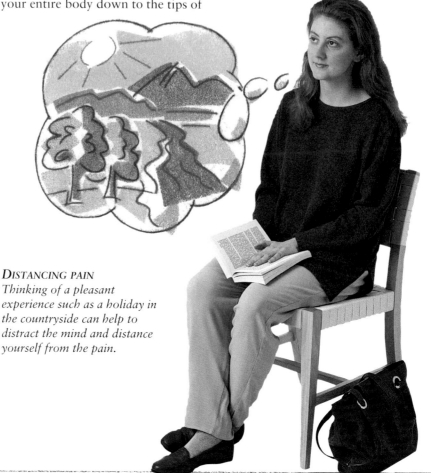

*DISTANCING PAIN*
*Thinking of a pleasant experience such as a holiday in the countryside can help to distract the mind and distance yourself from the pain.*

your toes and back up along the spine. Then imagine that the breath has reached the painful area and that when you exhale you are getting rid of the pain.

Practised correctly, a combination of visualisation and breathing techniques can relax you, help to conquer your fear and make a visit to a doctor a positive experience.

# PHOBIAS

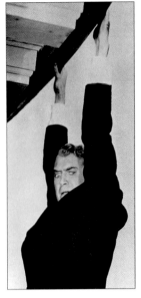

*FEAR OF HEIGHTS*
*One of the most famous fictional depictions of the obsessive behaviour of people suffering from phobias is in the film* Vertigo (1958). *The actor James Stewart plays a man who suffers from an irrational fear of heights after the woman he loves commits suicide by jumping off a tower.*

Phobias are irrational fears which can develop following sudden pain or shock. Some people may, for example, develop a fear of hospitals following a painful operation or an associated frightening experience as a child. Subsequently the feared situation will be avoided, so the fear is never confronted and tends to get worse. Other more generalised fears may then develop. Whenever the feared situation is experienced anxiety levels rise. If the situation is then immediately avoided the anxiety level will fall and the relief becomes associated with avoidance of the feared situation. If this happens repeatedly for a long period, conditioning can turn the fear into a phobia.

Fear of pain may mask a fear of something else. People will rationalise a fear, such as agoraphobia (fear of open spaces or entering public places), as being a fear of pain, because fear of physical pain is considered more understandable and therefore a more acceptable reason for not doing things than the apparently irrational fear. So, for example, a person might exaggerate a back pain as being so disabling as to prevent him or her from leaving the house, when in fact the underlying problem is psychological.

entails, how long it will last, what the side effects will be, what the long-term effects will be. Being informed will help you to feel in control, and in turn will make you feel less anxious. A recent UK study compared the levels of anxiety among terminally ill patients in institutions that had an open policy about discussing their patients' illnesses with those that had a policy of greater reticence. It found less anxiety and depression in the more open institutions.

## The importance of relaxation

After becoming well informed about your treatment and the pain you are likely to experience, the next most effective coping strategy is to learn how to relax. Relaxation can change your perception of pain, reducing its severity. The power of the mind over the body has been recognised since ancient times, but an interesting modern application of the phenomenon is demonstrated by the placebo effect.

The word placebo comes from Latin, meaning 'I please', and describes the use of a pill or other sham treatment, in place of a genuine painkiller or other active treatment. Although placebos are generally believed to be effective in cases of 'imaginary' pain, experiments now show that placebos can relieve actual physical symptoms related to diseases such as angina. According to research, an individual responds differently to placebos under different circumstances, at times responding and at others not. The exact way that placebos work is uncertain but the therapist's interest in the well-being of the patient, the patient's own belief that positive steps are being taken to relieve the pain and the consequent decrease in anxiety all seem to help contribute to a sense of relief and relaxation.

## Therapies for relaxation

A number of therapies are particularly effective at promoting relaxation. For example studies have shown that blood pressure, one of the indicators of stress and tension, drops during massage. Massage can also be very helpful in encouraging a good night's sleep, and sleep is perhaps the best form of natural healing and pain relief available.

Meditation is another extremely useful relaxation tool. Studies have shown that meditation can bring about a decreased heart rate, decreased respiration rate, decreased level of cortisol (a stress hormone) in the bloodstream, a lower pulse rate, and increased EEG (electro-encephalogram) alpha, a brain wave associated with relaxation. Defined simply, meditation refers to any activity that keeps your attention pleasantly focused in the present rather than dwelling on problems of the past or the future. Techniques to achieve this include exercises such as focusing the mind's attention on deep breathing to the exclusion of all other external stimuli. Many therapies also include a meditative aspect; for example, yoga, reiki and visualisation.

Chapter 4 describes in more detail relaxation techniques, energy-rebalancing and mind therapies that can all help to reduce anxiety and stress.

CHAPTER 2

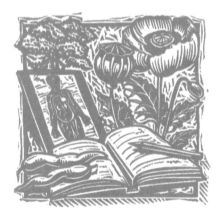

# PAIN AS A SYMPTOM

*Pain is the alarm bell of the body's sophisticated
signalling system, alerting us that something is
wrong. It serves not only to warn and protect, but
also to promote healing. Some types of pain can be
safely ignored or treated at home, while others
should be taken seriously and may warrant seeing
a doctor. An ability to distinguish between the
different types of pain will help you to decide
whether a visit to a doctor is advisable.*

# WARNING SIGNS

*Deciding when to call a doctor is not always easy. A knowledge of the different kinds of pain symptoms will make it easier to decipher any serious warning signs.*

If you learn to recognise different pain symptoms, you can begin to distinguish between pains you can manage yourself and pains that need to be treated by a doctor. In addition to helping you decide whether to visit a doctor, an understanding of your symptoms and an ability to describe them clearly and concisely will make it easier for your doctor to discover the cause of your pain and decide on the best possible course of treatment.

### LEARNING TO DISTINGUISH DIFFERENT KINDS OF PAIN

Many common aches and pains, such as headaches, muscle pain, indigestion, and cold hands and feet, usually do not signal any real threat to the body. The pain felt in these cases is caused by activation of the body's sensitive protective system by harmless stimuli, and although at times the pain may be strong, it does not indicate a serious problem and can usually be safely ignored. For example, women often feel pain during menstruation. This type of pain does not herald a major injury or disease, but is the body's reaction to hormones, which are released to stimulate the uterus to contract and shed its lining. These contractions can be very strong, causing severe cramps.

Sometimes the body's nervous system may break down and send faulty pain signals to the brain, resulting in chronic pain which has no meaningful purpose to its sufferer. An example of chronic pain is the prolonged discomfort which can follow a bout of shingles after the skin has healed and the virus causing the condition has been combated by medication or the body's own defences. Complementary medical techniques described in Chapter 4, such as massage and acupuncture, can help to alleviate chronic pain.

Sudden pain, such as the pain felt in the chest before a heart attack, serves as a true warning signal that the body is under threat and needs treatment. In such cases it is vital to consult a doctor as soon as possible.

### RECOGNISING THE WARNING SIGNS

Pain that signals a life-threatening condition is usually intense, starts abruptly, and is associated with other symptoms and signs. For example, a sudden severe headache accompanied by a fit, a feeling of weakness on one side of the body, or clouding of consciousness may signal acute brain haemorrhage. A chest pain that rapidly intensifies to unbearable levels, together with severe shortness of breath, dizziness or physical weakness, may indicate serious heart or lung disease. Acute abdominal pain accompanied by other major symptoms such as nausea, vomiting and signs of shock may indicate a perforated ulcer, inflammation of the pancreas, appendicitis or a similar condition requiring emergency surgery. Usually in such cases, the severity of the pain clearly tells a person that their symptoms are not trivial and they need to seek help.

### DEALING WITH GRADUAL PAIN

In many cases pain comes on gradually, slowly building to a point at which it interferes with daily life and you need to take action. It may arise as a discomfort which slowly turns into an actual pain that does not abate. Or it may result from an injury or another easily detectable cause such as period cramps, over-strenuous exercise, bruising, or indigestion. In such circumstances you will probably decide to treat your own pain, and if you use common sense this should be quite sufficient. There are a variety of home remedies that can be safely used to treat common painful ailments such as period pains, indigestion, headaches and coughs (see table opposite).

*SHINGLES CELLS*
*The most excruciating pain in shingles can occur after the blisters have healed, because the virus may remain in some nerves. Part of an infected cell is shown in yellow in the lower right corner of the picture.*

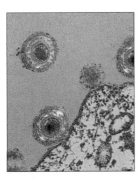

Two extremely effective treatments for various types of common pain, such as sprains and rheumatic aches, are heating and cooling. However, it is important to distinguish between their uses. Cooling should be used to treat the inflammation caused by strains and sprains. It soothes the skin and helps to neutralise the release of chemicals in the damaged tissue, such as prostaglandins, that cause inflammation and pain. However, an icepack should only be used to soothe very painful and highly inflamed injuries as it can inhibit the healing process.

Warming is effective for chronic pain such as aching joints caused by rheumatism. Warming the damaged area stimulates the pain receptors further, so that even more pain messages are transmitted to the brain. As a result the pain gate becomes overloaded and no further pain messages can be interpreted. Stimulating the skin also helps to relax the underlying muscles.

In some cases a judicious mix of warming and cooling techniques, for example by using hot then cold compresses, or alternate hot and cold baths can also be beneficial. Pain-relieving sprays which are often used by physiotherapists for the first-aid treatment of sports injuries have a longer-lasting effect than superficially cooling the skin. For further information on how to make and apply a compress see pages 87 and 155.

## HOME REMEDIES

Some types of pain can be safely treated at home without the need for prescribed medical painkillers. In many cases, such as a sprain or period pain, applying heat or a cold compress can be extremely effective.

Simple measures such as herbal remedies or gentle exercise may also provide relief in some situations. But if pain persists after treatment with a home remedy you should consult a doctor for further advice.

| PAIN | TREATMENT | AIM | METHOD | WARNING |
|---|---|---|---|---|
| Rheumatic aches | Heat | Soothes soft tissue and causes counter-irritation | Hot-water bottle; hot compress; rheumatic liniment and spray | Don't use in cases of flare-up of existing symptoms |
| | Pressure | Relaxes tense muscles and causes counter-irritation | Acupressure; gentle massage | |
| Strains and sprains | Cooling | Reduces inflammation by neutralising prostaglandins in damaged tissue | Cooling spray, pack of frozen peas; apply for 10 mins, re-apply 1 hour later | Wrap ice pack in a towel to prevent iceburn |
| | Rest | Reduces swelling | Raise injured part | |
| Headache | Over-the-counter painkillers; herbal remedies | Reduces inflammation; blocks pain; relaxes muscles | Take recommended dose with water | If headaches persist consult your doctor |
| | Relaxation | Reduces nervous tension | Rest in the dark; massage temples; relax in a hot bath | |
| Period pains | Heat | Reduces muscle spasm | Take a hot bath; apply a hot sponge or hot-water bottle | If pain persists after menstruation see a doctor |
| | Gentle exercise | Stimulates release of endorphins; relaxes muscles | Go for a bicycle ride; go swimming; take a walk | |
| Indigestion | Herbal remedies and antacids | Neutralises stomach acid and soothes inflammation of stomach lining | Take milk, yoghurt after meals; drink camomile or peppermint tea | If indigestion is persistent or recurrent, see your doctor |

## LOCATING THE LIKELY CAUSE OF PAIN

The human skin contains an intricate network of nerve endings which accurately locate the site and nature of any painful stimulus. For example, if you cut your finger then pain is felt on your finger at the site of the injury. However, other organs are not as well supplied with nerve endings and so the exact location and cause of pain, say in the abdomen, is more difficult to pinpoint.

Furthermore, many pain messages are bundled together and transmitted along a common nerve pathway. This may result in the brain misinterpreting a pain message as coming from a different part of the body. In such cases pain is felt at another site, sometimes in a completely different area from the original injury (see page 21). This is known as 'referred pain'. For example, pain felt in the mid-back can actually be a warning signal of problems in the pancreas in the abdominal cavity. Determining the originating site of and reason for a pain can therefore require considerable skill and is best trusted to professionals.

## THE LOCATION OF YOUR PAIN

To understand the nature of your pain, it's important to remember that pain felt in certain parts of the body might be referred from an injury in another part of the body.

Jaw, neck and throat pain may be due to problems in the **jaw joint**

Pain in the forehead and behind the eye may be referred from problems in the **neck**

Right upper abdomen and right shoulder pain may indicate problems in the **gall bladder**

Pain in the chest wall, arm, throat or jaw may be an indicator of **heart** problems

Pain in the upper abdomen, mid-back and shoulder blade may be due to problems in the **pancreas**

Upper abdomen and mid-back pain may indicate problems in the **stomach**

Pain in the side of the abdomen may be referred from problems in the **kidneys**

Pain in the lower abdomen may be caused by problems in the **bladder**

Pain in the leg may indicate problems in the **spinal cord**

## SEEKING HELP FROM NATURAL THERAPISTS

Aches and pains are often relieved by massage, acupuncture, chiropractic treatment, osteopathy, relaxation therapies and other natural techniques. As treatments they have variable outcomes, and different individuals may show remarkably different responses to them. With proper precautions these treatments are safe and are increasingly popular.

However, it's important to remember that complementary medicine does not always show immediate results so don't expect a miracle cure. Although starting a new treatment can make you feel optimistic about a cure, the realisation that a technique is not working for you can lead to depression, which in turn can heighten your perception of pain. Some treatments, such as acupuncture, chiropractic and transcutaneous nerve stimulation (TENS) may even cause additional pain initially, but in the longer term they can help alleviate the pain associated with chronic diseases. Unless you suffer from frequent recurrence of an old condition, you should see your doctor first. This is especially important if your pain features any of the warning symptoms (see page 38).

### Combining natural therapies with medical treatment

Complementary medical treatment is commonly used with orthodox medicine. For example, you might try aromatherapy and hydrotherapy in conjunction with medical painkillers to help to relieve migraine pain.

Natural remedies are generally safe if you follow a few simple guidelines. Always let your doctor know what additional methods you intend to try, so that if necessary your medical treatment can be adjusted accordingly. You should also tell your doctor if you are using herbal medicines as they could interfere with drug treatment. If you are receiving physiotherapy, the practitioner should be made aware of any treatment by an osteopath or chiropractor, so that practices do not overlap.

Conversely, some complementary practitioners express concern that their treatment may not be as effective if you are also using drugs prescribed by a doctor. However, you should not stop taking prescribed medication without consulting your doctor. For more information on complementary medicines and their uses see Chapter 4.

# THE MCGILL PAIN QUESTIONNAIRE

The McGill pain questionnaire was originally developed as a research tool at McGill University in Montreal, Canada. Ronald Melzack, one of the world's top pain researchers, compiled a list of common words used by pain sufferers to describe their pain. Doctors then started to give the words to patients to help them describe their own symptoms.

To use the questionnaire, look carefully through the 20 groups of words. If a word in any group applies to your pain, circle that word. Do not circle more than one word in a group. If there are groups of words that do not apply to your pain, there is no need to circle a word. Then go over the circled words in groups 1 to 10 and choose the three that most closely represent your pain and write them down. Similarly, choose the two most representative circled words from groups 11 to 15. Write down the one circled word in group 16, and one word chosen from the remaining groups 17 to 20.

You should end up with up to seven words that describe the quality and intensity of your pain and give an indication of how it affects you. These words should help your therapist to assess the impact of your pain on your well-being and then to plan a possible course of treatment to try to alleviate it.

| GROUP 1 | GROUP 2 | GROUP 3 | GROUP 4 |
|---|---|---|---|
| Flickering | Jumping | Pricking | Sharp |
| Quivering | Flashing | Boring | Gritting |
| Pulsing | Shooting | Drilling | Lacerating |
| Throbbing | | Stabbing | |
| Beating | | | |
| Pounding | | | |

| GROUP 5 | GROUP 6 | GROUP 7 | GROUP 8 |
|---|---|---|---|
| Pinching | Tugging | Hot | Tingling |
| Pressing | Pulling | Burning | Itching |
| Gnawing | Wrenching | Scalding | Smarting |
| Cramping | | Searing | Stinging |
| Crushing | | | |

| GROUP 9 | GROUP 10 | GROUP 11 | GROUP 12 |
|---|---|---|---|
| Dull | Tender | Tiring | Sickening |
| Sore | Taut | Exhausting | Suffocating |
| Hurting | Rasping | | |
| Aching | Splitting | | |
| Heavy | | | |

| GROUP 13 | GROUP 14 | GROUP 15 | GROUP 16 |
|---|---|---|---|
| Fearful | Punishing | Wretched | Annoying |
| Frightful | Gruelling | Blinding | Troublesome |
| Terrifying | Cruel | | Miserable |
| | Vicious | | Intense |
| | Killing | | Unbearable |

| GROUP 17 | GROUP 18 | GROUP 19 | GROUP 20 |
|---|---|---|---|
| Spreading | Tight | Cool | Nagging |
| Radiating | Numb | Cold | Nauseating |
| Penetrating | Drawing | Freezing | Agonising |
| Piercing | Squeezing | | Dreadful |
| | Tearing | | Torturing |

# The GP

*Building a good relationship with your local GP is an important step in the successful management of pain. The following guidelines show you how careful preparation can help your GP to diagnose your problem and suggest appropriate treatment.*

## Origins

Health care is one of the oldest professions. In medieval times apothecaries, or pharmacists, used their knowledge of herbal medicine to cure sick members of the community. Their modern equivalent is the GP, or general practitioner. Before the Second World War, GPs mostly operated alone from their own homes. However, after 1945 GPs started to form partnerships with other doctors and today's purpose-built surgeries are well equipped and staffed by teams of qualified nurses and clerical staff.

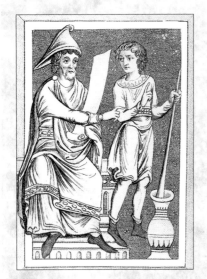

*ANCIENT TRADITIONS*
*Medieval medicine was based on a knowledge of herbal lore that had been handed down for centuries.*

When it is time to visit your doctor, it pays to be prepared. A body chart indicating the location of your pain, a pain diary (see page 44) describing your pain in detail, and a daily record of the intensity of your pain will help your doctor to diagnose the cause of your pain and suggest appropriate treatment. It is also a good idea to rehearse what you plan to say to the doctor to make sure your description is accurate and complete: although you need to be concise, it is important not to miss out details which may be relevant to the doctor's diagnosis.

### Does my doctor need to know exactly where the pain is?

Yes. A body chart showing the precise location of your pain or pains is extremely helpful in giving your doctor a good idea at a glance. It's particularly important to keep a body chart if the site of your pain varies, such as in the case of a migraine. Do not clutter the chart with detailed information, but try to concentrate only on the main issues. Your doctor can always form a more detailed picture to pinpoint your pain by asking you for more information.

### I find it difficult to explain my pain. Any suggestions?

Many people find it helpful to follow the McGill pain questionnaire (see page 41), which can help to pin down the particular nature of your pain. The questionnaire was originally developed for use in

research and has been translated into many languages. The questionnaire lists 77 words chosen from those most commonly used by patients to describe their pain. The first ten groups of words describe the quality of pain, groups 11 to 15 describe how the pain affects you, group 16 evaluates the intensity of the pain, and the rest are miscellaneous.

### How can the doctor measure my pain?

You can help the doctor to get a picture of its intensity and its fluctuations by measuring your pain yourself. One system of measurement is the visual analogue scale (VAS), which you can easily make at home (see right). By marking the intensity of your pain on a blank scale every day, changes in the degree of pain felt over a period of time can be detected. Prepare several VAS scales so that you can record the intensity of your pain once or even twice a day for a given period, say over a week or two. Every day try to make time to mark the point that you think represents the level of your pain, then write the date and time on the scale so you can track any fluctuations. It's important that you don't look at previous recordings before making your mark on the line. Although a VAS report can help your doctor to understand your pain, remember that it is subjective and relates only to your own experience. It is not possible to compare pain reports from different people, as individuals have different perceptions and experiences of pain.

## Does my doctor have time to go over all this information?

Your doctor will be able to grasp the essence of your pain quickly if you have your pain scales and pain diary to hand. He or she will then be able to devote more time to examining you and planning investigations and treatment. Your doctor will probably ask you to carry on recording your pain in the same way so that it is possible to monitor whether the treatment is working.

## Why can't I just ask the doctor to investigate what is wrong with me?

Remember that pain is a personal and subjective experience – your doctor cannot actually 'see' your pain. The doctor has to rely on your description of your pain in order to decide on appropriate treatment. It is best to do all that you can to convey information about your pain precisely and concisely. If you are not able to record notes and pain charts, one way to describe your pain is to imagine what you would have to do to someone to cause that

---

## MAKE YOUR OWN VISUAL ANALOGUE SCALE

Draw a line on a piece of paper and divide it into ten equal sections. At one end write 'No pain at all' and at the other write 'The worst pain I ever felt'. Now put a cross on the scale to represent your current level of pain. Prepare enough scales to use a new one each time so that you're not influenced by previous recordings (for more details, see opposite). A similar scale can be used to record the effectiveness of different types of painkiller – at one end write the name of the drug and the time you took it. Mark on the scale the length of time that you are pain-free. This will help the doctor to adjust the dosage correctly.

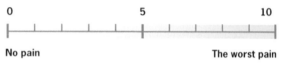

**0**          **5**          **10**

**No pain**                **The worst pain**

*PAIN GAUGE*
*Record your pain at the same time each day.*

---

kind of pain. Thrust a dagger between the shoulder blades and twist it? Tie a belt around the head and pull it tight? After forming as clear a picture as possible of what you are feeling, the doctor can then start planning your treatment.

## Can the doctor advise me about long-term treatment?

To plan your treatment programme and remain in control of it, you need to have as much information as possible about the options available. If your GP suggests new treatment

always ask for a clear explanation of what is going to happen and about any possible risks. Your GP can help you to interpret any data you may have from journals or specialist groups. He or she can also advise about the possibility of combining orthodox medical treatment with complementary approaches such as chiropractors, osteopaths, pain clinics, healers and self-help groups. Many GPs have been trained in complementary health care and some practices include complementary practitioners on the staff.

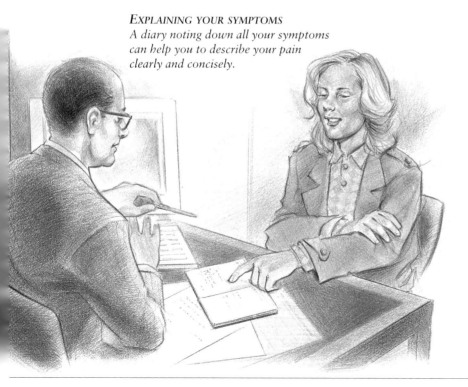

*EXPLAINING YOUR SYMPTOMS*
*A diary noting down all your symptoms can help you to describe your pain clearly and concisely.*

## WHAT YOU CAN DO AT HOME

Before a visit to the GP go over in your mind how you are going to explain your pain symptoms to the doctor. Use this checklist to make sure you have everything you need to support your description:

▶ *Pain diary (see page 44).*

▶ *VAS scales measuring the intensity of pain (see above and opposite).*

▶ *List of words describing your pain (see page 41).*

▶ *Notebook and pen to write down advice and prescription details.*

▶ *Details of medication and its effects.*

*Keeping a*

# Pain Diary

*Pain, particularly chronic pain, is notoriously difficult to describe, but your doctor or complementary health practitioner needs a clear description in order to determine the possible causes for your condition and suggest appropriate treatment.*

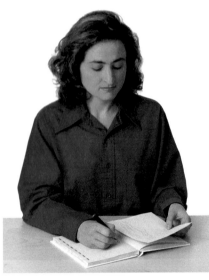

**GETTING TO GRIPS WITH YOUR PAIN**
*A good way of forming a clearer picture of the nature of your pain is to record your symptoms in a pain diary.*

By making a careful daily record of what you are feeling, you will start to reach a clearer understanding of the type of pain you suffer – its nature, intensity and fluctuations. Note down your pain in a diary alongside events in your daily life; this should give you a good idea of any factors that make your pain worse, such as stress, as well as conditions that help to ease the pain, such as a good night's sleep. This knowledge will help your therapist to choose a suitable form of treatment and to suggest ways of avoiding such pain in future.

**The amount of pain** and whether the pain started abruptly or gradually may be important factors in assessing your condition.

**Words from the McGill pain questionnaire** can help your therapist to understand the particular quality of your pain.

**The painkillers you take and their effects** should be recorded so that your therapist can check your progress.

**Changes in the nature of your pain** and whether the pain is constant or intermittent can be highly significant in the correct diagnosis of your condition. Note how long each bout lasts.

**Stressful events** that may influence the onset of your pain should be carefully noted down.

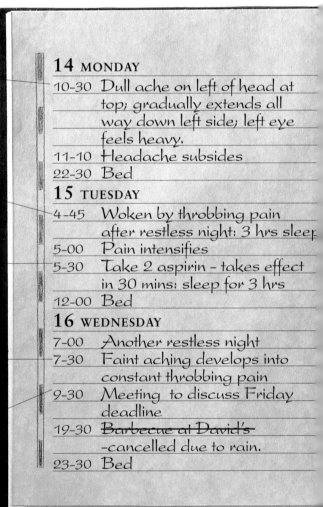

**14** MONDAY

10-30  Dull ache on left of head at top; gradually extends all way down left side; left eye feels heavy.

11-10  Headache subsides

22-30  Bed

**15** TUESDAY

4-45  Woken by throbbing pain after restless night: 3 hrs sleep

5-00  Pain intensifies

5-30  Take 2 aspirin – takes effect in 30 mins: sleep for 3 hrs

12-00  Bed

**16** WEDNESDAY

7-00  Another restless night

7-30  Faint aching develops into constant throbbing pain

9-30  Meeting to discuss Friday deadline

19-30  ~~Barbecue at David's~~ –cancelled due to rain.

23-30  Bed

A clear description of your pain is particularly important in the diagnosis of conditions such as migraine and irritable bowel syndrome. These conditions may not be characterised by any obvious physical abnormality and so the doctor or health practitioner's diagnosis depends heavily on an accurate pain description. Also, a pain diary will help you and your doctor to see the patterns of your pain. This is useful in conditions such as migraine, gallstones, kidney stones, gout and angina, as these often feature recurrent pain attacks.

The diary gives a solid account of your pain for the doctor or health practitioner to review and provides further leads to follow as required. He or she may also ask about your mood, appetite, personal relations and work, especially if the pain is chronic. All this information has a bearing on the distress you feel, and helps to determine what type of investigations and treatment you should undergo.

If you are taking any medication, you may find it useful to keep a record of the type, dosage, its results and any side effects so that your doctor can monitor your treatment.

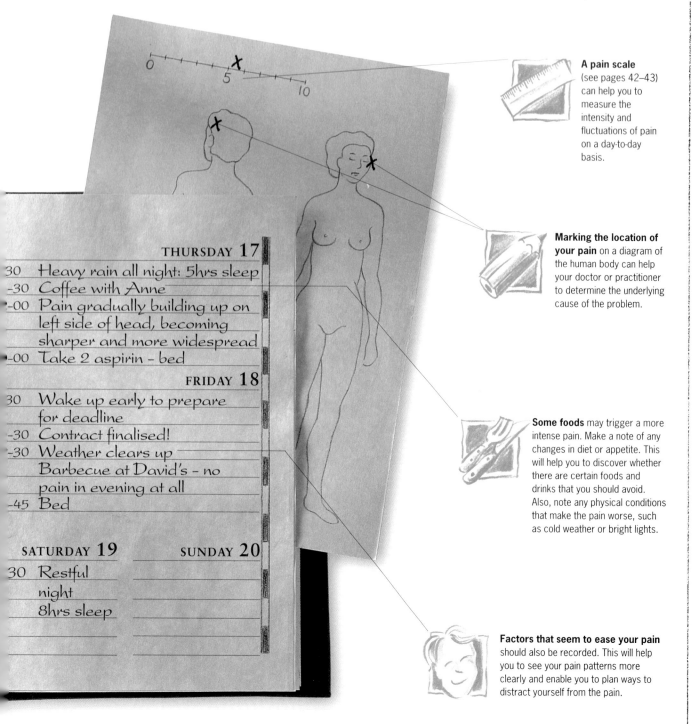

**A pain scale** (see pages 42–43) can help you to measure the intensity and fluctuations of pain on a day-to-day basis.

**Marking the location of your pain** on a diagram of the human body can help your doctor or practitioner to determine the underlying cause of the problem.

**Some foods** may trigger a more intense pain. Make a note of any changes in diet or appetite. This will help you to discover whether there are certain foods and drinks that you should avoid. Also, note any physical conditions that make the pain worse, such as cold weather or bright lights.

**Factors that seem to ease your pain** should also be recorded. This will help you to see your pain patterns more clearly and enable you to plan ways to distract yourself from the pain.

**THURSDAY 17**

30 Heavy rain all night: 5hrs sleep
-30 Coffee with Anne
-00 Pain gradually building up on left side of head, becoming sharper and more widespread
-00 Take 2 aspirin - bed

**FRIDAY 18**

30 Wake up early to prepare for deadline
-30 Contract finalised!
-30 Weather clears up Barbecue at David's - no pain in evening at all
-45 Bed

**SATURDAY 19**          **SUNDAY 20**

30 Restful night 8hrs sleep

# PAINKILLERS

*A variety of natural and orthodox painkillers are available that can help to relieve most pains. Whether bought over the counter or prescribed by a doctor, they should all be used with care.*

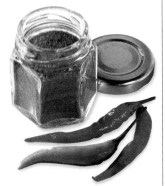

**VERSATILE SPICE**
*The versatile medicinal uses of cayenne pepper have long been known to American natives. The spice contains the painkilling ingredient capsaicin that can be used internally, to ease toothache for example, or externally, in a poultice for joint pain.*

Natural and orthodox painkillers can be used to relieve a variety of pains ranging from mild toothache to the chest pains of a heart attack. Both natural and orthodox painkillers are available over the counter at pharmacies.

In general, natural painkillers are more effective at alleviating pain in the long term than giving immediate relief. As they cause relatively few side effects, it is quite safe to use natural painkillers over an extended period to relieve pain and help prevent recurrence of painful symptoms. (Their use is further explored in the section on herbalism on page 86.)

Conversely, orthodox painkillers are fast-acting, having an effect soon after they are taken. However, it is not safe to take medical painkillers in the long term as they may cause undesirable side effects such as bleeding in the stomach and liver damage. If you have been taking over-the-counter pain-killers such as aspirin or paracetamol for 48 hours and the symptoms still persist, you should consult a doctor as soon as possible. The doctor will be able to advise on further treatment, which might include stronger drugs available only on prescription.

### NATURAL PAINKILLERS
The healing properties of plants and herbs have been recognised since ancient times. It has been estimated that even today the majority of the world's population relies on natural medicines for treatment of aches and pains, and it is often forgotten that many of today's orthodox painkillers are derived from plants. For example, aspirin is derived from the bark of the white willow and morphine from the unripe seed pods of the opium poppy. Natural painkillers can be particularly effective at relieving the pain of common ailments such as rheumatism, headache, and damage to nerves.

## NATURAL PAINKILLERS

A variety of natural ingredients can be used to relieve a range of painful disorders. Many of these natural painkillers consist of kitchen herbs that are easily grown at home. For more information on the use of natural painkillers for specific conditions see Chapters 5 to 8. For more information on herbalism see page 86.

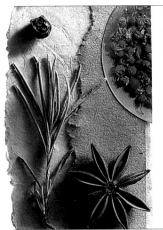

| PAIN | NATURAL PAINKILLER | TREATMENT |
|------|--------------------|-----------|
| Rheumatic pain | Camphor from *Cinnamomum camphora*<br>Camomile from *Chamaemelum nobilis* | Apply camphor oil to painful area; drink camomile tea<br>Take in tablet form or drink tea made from leaves |
| Chilblains | Wintergreen from *Gaultheria procumbens*<br>(pure oil may cause an allergic reaction) | Make poultice from leaves and apply to chilblain, or soak cloth in wintergreen oil and place on chilblain |
| Migraine | Feverfew (*Chrysanthemum parthenicum*)<br>Lavender (*Lavandula angustifolia*)<br>Capsaicin from *Capsicum frutescens* | Drink tea made from fresh or dried feverfew leaves<br>Drink tea made from lavender flowers<br>Take capsaicin internally in powder or in tablet form |
| Cramps | Cramp bark (*Viburnum opulus*)<br>Rosemary (*Rosemarinus officinalis*) | Drink tea made from bark<br>Apply rosemary oil externally |
| Indigestion | Peppermint (*Mentha piperita*) | Drink tea made from mint leaves |

Natural products are widely available from chemists, health food shops and many supermarkets in a variety of forms. Dried herbs such as peppermint and sage can be used not only to make infusions for drinking but also in poultices for placing directly over a painful area. Infusions of lavender and feverfew are well-tested alternatives to orthodox medical painkillers for treating headaches and migraines.

Cayenne pepper or chilli pepper contains capsaicin which causes the hot tingling feeling in the mouth when pepper is eaten. This feeling is brought about because capsaicin first stimulates 'C' fibres (slow-conducting fibres) but then deactivates them so that pain messages are effectively prevented from reaching the brain. Capsaicin is widely used to treat a variety of ailments such as nerve damage and stomach cramps, and as a general tonic. It can also be used externally in a poultice to ease the pain of rheumatism and arthritis. In addition, various natural oils are available which can be massaged into the skin to soothe pain by causing the pain gate to close to further pain messages. Pain caused by aching arthritic joints can often be soothed by massaging the affected area with cajaput oil from the white tea tree.

Natural painkillers are usually kinder to the body than orthodox painkillers because they have relatively few side effects. It's important to remember, however, that natural painkillers may sometimes take longer to become effective, and so are probably better suited to relieving chronic pain rather than acute pain.

If your pain persists after using a home herbal remedy, you could try consulting a registered medical herbalist for a full assessment and prescription (see Chapter 4).

### ORTHODOX PAINKILLERS

Orthodox painkillers give immediate pain relief, but should be used with caution in the long term because of the danger of serious side effects such as gastric bleeding and liver damage. A knowledge of the workings and effects of these painkillers can help you to plan your treatment. Orthodox painkillers can be broadly divided into two groups: non-narcotic and narcotic drugs.

Non-narcotic painkillers, except for paracetamol, are similar in effect to aspirin and are effective for relieving mild pain and reducing inflammation.

## Origins

The common painkiller we know as aspirin is actually derived from a plant, white willow (*Salix alba*). It has been known for its ability to relieve pain since Roman times. The healing properties of its leaves and bark were first brought to the attention of the medical world in modern times when an English clergyman wrote to the Royal Society in 1763 about his success at treating rheumatic fevers with willow. In the early 19th century, scientists succeeded in isolating the active substance from willow bark and called it salicin. In 1899 Heinrich Dreser (1860–1925) discovered acetylsalicylic acid, a compound derived from salicin, which caused relatively few side-effects. The drug was marketed under the name 'Aspirin'.

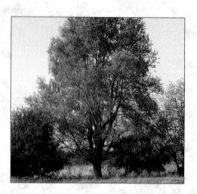

**WHITE WILLOW**
*In ancient times the leaves or bark were crushed in olive oil and applied externally.*

Almost all narcotic painkillers are related to morphine which is derived from opium and include such drugs as codeine. These are used for treating more severe pain.

### NON-NARCOTIC DRUGS

Non-narcotic painkillers are mild and are used for treating moderate pains such as flu symptoms, headaches, muscle cramps and toothache. Non-narcotic drugs include paracetamol and the non-steroidal anti-inflammatory drugs (NSAIDs) such as ibuprofen and aspirin. For more severe pain a combination of non-narcotic drugs, such as aspirin or paracetamol, and narcotic drugs, such as codeine, is commonly prescribed.

## How non-narcotic drugs work

If the body is injured or infected, chemicals known as prostaglandins are released. These chemicals trigger the transmission of pain messages to the brain and encourage inflammation of the damaged area. Non-narcotic painkillers (except paracetamol) block the production of these chemicals, thus preventing pain signals from being produced, and stopping the pain while reducing inflammation. However, inflammation is not stopped completely so the healing process can continue. Paracetamol

## DO'S AND DON'TS OF TAKING PAINKILLERS

When using painkillers, follow the instructions carefully to maximise the benefits and minimise the side effects.

▶ *Never take more than the recommended dosage.*

▶ *Don't use more than one over-the-counter painkiller at a time. They may contain similar ingredients which could lead to an overdose.*

▶ *Tell your doctor if you use over-the-counter drugs, as there may be drug interactions.*

▶ *Consult your doctor before taking painkillers if you have an ulcer or history of liver or kidney disease.*

▶ *Take with water or, for quicker absorption, half a cup of coffee or tea.*

▶ *Beware: some people feel drowsy after taking painkillers. If you are affected, don't drive.*

*EASY RELIEF*
*Take painkillers with water while sitting or standing so they don't become stuck in your gullet.*

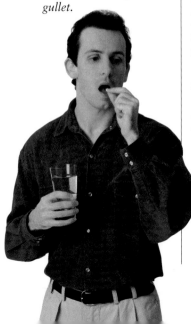

# HOW PAINKILLERS WORK

Non-narcotics (with the exception of paracetamol) and narcotics have quite a different painkilling action. Non-narcotics are effective at controlling inflammation because they act at the site of injury, while narcotics (and paracetamol) relieve pain by stopping pain messages at the dorsal horn.

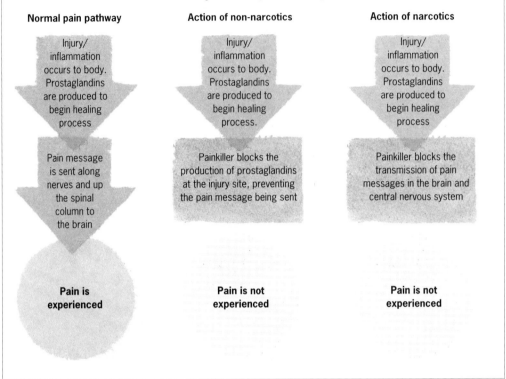

**Normal pain pathway**

Injury/inflammation occurs to body. Prostaglandins are produced to begin healing process

Pain message is sent along nerves and up the spinal column to the brain

**Pain is experienced**

**Action of non-narcotics**

Injury/inflammation occurs to body. Prostaglandins are produced to begin healing process.

Painkiller blocks the production of prostaglandins at the injury site, preventing the pain message being sent

**Pain is not experienced**

**Action of narcotics**

Injury/inflammation occurs to body. Prostaglandins are produced to begin healing process

Painkiller blocks the transmission of pain messages in the brain and central nervous system

**Pain is not experienced**

is also a mild painkiller but does not effect the release of prostaglandins or reduce inflammation. It is believed to work by blocking the transmission of pain messages in the brain and central nervous system.

## Aspirin

Aspirin is a mild non-narcotic painkiller used to relieve moderate pains such as headaches and period pains. It also helps to reduce inflammation so it may be prescribed for joint pain, such as arthritis.

Aspirin can cause stomach upsets and nausea but these unpleasant side effects can be avoided by using coated tablets which dissolve lower down in the intestine. If you take aspirin over two days and it fails to relieve the pain, you should consult a doctor. Use of aspirin over a long period is not advisable as it can cause bleeding in the stomach. You should not give aspirin to children except under medical supervision because there is a slight risk of a rare disorder called Reye's syndrome, which can involve severe brain and liver damage.

## Other non-steroidal anti-inflammatory drugs (NSAIDs)

NSAIDs are widely used to relieve pain, reduce inflammation and lower body temperature. They include the drugs diclofenac and ibuprofen. They are particularly effective at reducing inflammation of muscles and joints caused by arthritis and gout.

Although NSAIDs take effect quickly, they can cause unpleasant side effects. Gastric irritation is common, particularly if the drugs are used over a long period of time. You can minimise the risk of side effects from NSAIDs by using them for a short period of time only and by taking them with food and milk. Although the possibility of side effects from NSAIDs can vary widely according to the patient, ibuprofen has been shown to cause the least amount of gastric discomfort. NSAIDs can also cause rashes, dizziness and tinnitus, and, in rare cases, damage to the liver or kidneys. If you experience abdominal pain after taking NSAIDs you should ask your doctor for advice on an alternative drug.

## Paracetamol

Paracetamol is a simple painkiller suitable for mild aches and pains. It is particularly recommended for people who suffer frequent stomach upsets, because unlike aspirin and other NSAIDs, paracetamol doesn't cause stomach problems. It is also safe for children to take provided it is given at the correct dosage. It is available as a syrup to use in treating children. However, because it doesn't inhibit prostaglandins, it doesn't reduce inflammation. It is therefore not as effective as aspirin for treating arthritis, or injuries to soft tissue such as muscles and ligaments.

If you take paracetamol, read the instructions and never exceed the recommended dosage. It is highly toxic in large doses: as few as 20 tablets can cause fatal liver damage. However, if taken in the recommended dosage it has few side effects. If you have a weak liver, an alternative is the more expensive paracetamol formulation containing an antidote to its possible toxic effects.

### NARCOTIC DRUGS

Weak narcotics such as codeine and dextropropoxyphene are used to treat cases of moderate pain. For example, codeine is used in cough medicines and some anti-diarrhoea medications. Weak narcotics cause a heightened feeling of excitement and if patients use them over a long period of time, they have a tendency to demand larger doses. However, if the recommended dosage is taken over a limited period there is little danger of them becoming addictive.

Strong narcotics such as diamorphine, morphine, pethidine and pentazosine are used to relieve the severe pain caused by serious injury, major surgery or in chronic disease when other painkillers have proved ineffective. However, they are not so effective in treating nerve pain. This is usually because substances produced in damaged nerves prevent their action or because the nerve receptors themselves are damaged so that narcotics can't switch them on to help in the blocking of pain stimuli.

## MEDICAL PAINKILLERS

Some medical painkillers are available over the counter at pharmacies (indicated below with an asterisk); others are only on prescription. The first five drugs listed below are examples of non-narcotics while the others are classed as narcotics. If you experience any unpleasant side effects, consult your doctor.

| DRUG | TIME TO TAKE EFFECT | SINGLE ADULT DOSE | MAX PER DAY | SIDE EFFECTS AND COMMENTS |
|---|---|---|---|---|
| Paracetamol* | ½–1 hour | 500–1000 mg 4–6 hrs | 4000 mg | Safe for children, pregnant women and asthmatics but not for those with liver disease; high risk of overdose |
| Aspirin* | ½–2 hours | 300–900 mg 4–6 hours | 4000 mg | Gastric irritation; stomach bleeding and ulcers; tinnitus; Reyes syndrome (children) |
| Ibuprofen* | ½–1 hour | 200–400 mg 6–8 hours | 2400 mg | Few side effects: indigestion; stomach ulcers; confusion in elderly |
| Diclofenac | 2 hours | 50 mg 8–12 hours | 150 mg | Indigestion; stomach ulcers; confusion in elderly; rash |
| Naproxen | 2–3 hours | 500 mg (initially) 6–8 hrs | 1250 mg | Indigestion; stomach ulcers; confusion in elderly |
| Codeine | ½–1 hour | 30–60 mg every 4 hours | 240 mg | Constipation; nausea; mildly addictive |
| D-propoxy-phene | ½–2 hours | 65 mg every 6–8 hours | 260 mg | Sedation; constipation; nausea; mildly addictive |
| Morphine | ½–1 hour | 10–30 mg 4 hours | Not applicable | Sedation; constipation; itching; risk of addiction |

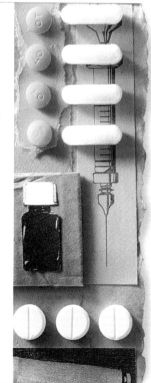

## Origins

Opium, a strong painkiller, is derived from the seed pods of a particular species of poppy, *Papaver somniferum*. It has been known since ancient times as an effective pain reliever – the Sumerians used it to soothe colicky children and the Romans used it to cure a range of painful symptoms. Opium is also known for its ability to create a pleasant euphoric state. Since the last century, pharmacologists have attempted to modify opium to produce substances which are longer-lasting, or have a shorter and more intense effect. The most well known of these drugs are heroin and morphine, which played a major part in the advancement of medical science in the 19th century because of their ability to relieve severe pain, such as that experienced after major surgery.

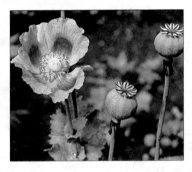

PAPAVER SOMNIFERUM
*The first regular use of opium was in the Far East where it was either smoked or eaten.*

Patients taking strong narcotics experience drowsiness, mood swings and impaired mental activity in addition to very effective pain relief. Unpleasant side effects, such as nausea, constipation and itching, are also common. As patients may become dependent on these drugs, they cannot be used over a long period.

### How narcotic drugs work

Narcotic drugs are powerful painkillers. Unlike NSAIDs, which block pain messages at the site of an injury, narcotics work within the brain and central nervous system to prevent the transmission of pain signals. Narcotic drugs combine at specific sites known as opiate receptors located in the spinal cord and mid-brain to block the transmission of pain signals to the brain, thereby preventing the perception of pain.

Unfortunately, however, opiate receptors are also located at various sites all over the body, so when narcotic drugs are injected, this not only achieves the desired pain relief but also results in other physiological effects. Some of these may be beneficial, particularly those in the nervous system, where the drugs produce a marked reduction in anxiety. Other side effects may be undesirable however, such as nausea, constipation and potential addiction.

### Antidepressants and anticonvulsants

You may be surprised to find that your doctor prescribes antidepressants for nerve pain or similar disorders. These drugs are usually used to treat mood disorders, but they are also effective in relieving pain. They can help to improve sleep, which is often disturbed in chronic pain sufferers. However, antidepressants do not provide fast pain relief: they generally take two to three weeks, and for the peak effect four to six weeks. In addition their use is often associated with a dry mouth and constipation, although some of these side effects may diminish over time. Not all antidepressant drugs have this pain-relieving property – the exceptions include some very common antidepressants such as fluoxetine (Prozac).

Anticonvulsants, commonly used to treat epilepsy, are also effective in treating certain types of nerve pain, especially sharp, shooting pains. They act on the nerve fibres and prevent them from firing pain messages without cause. Both antidepressants and anticonvulsants are effective only if used on a continual basis. Although antidepressants are not addictive, patients often suffer side effects such as drowsiness, dizziness and memory impairment which reflect the action of the drugs on the processes of the nervous system.

### Corticosteroid drugs

Corticosteroids are a group of powerful drugs related to natural hormones produced in the body. They are effective at reducing inflammation and so are often used to relieve intestinal disorders such as Crohn's disease (see page 112) and inflamed tendons and joints caused by such conditions as tennis elbow (see page 137). Corticosteroids act by reducing the production of prostaglandins and suppressing the immune system. Because of their potency, they should be used with extreme caution.

#### LONG-TERM DRUG TREATMENT

In the short term, drugs may provide relief from pain. However, for chronic pain many people choose to avoid the unpleasant side effects of conventional drugs by trying alternative therapies (see Chapter 4). As well as helping to reduce the pain, many of these therapies use manipulative techniques, or suggest dietary and other lifestyle changes that may treat the underlying cause.

# CHAPTER 3

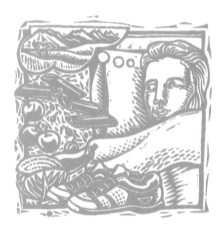

# STRATEGIES FOR PREVENTING PAIN

*The pain caused by some illnesses, especially
stress-related diseases, can in many cases be avoided
by looking after your mind and body. An active
and responsible attitude towards your health, in
partnership with your doctor and other health
practitioners, is the first step towards preventing a
whole range of painful symptoms.*

# IMPROVING YOUR LIFESTYLE

*A stressful job, poor diet, incorrect posture and lack of exercise can all influence the onset of painful disorders. Improving your lifestyle may help you to avoid pain and illness in the future.*

## GETTING A GOOD NIGHT'S SLEEP

There are several ways you can help yourself to a good night's sleep:

▶ *Cut down on coffee and tea and other drinks which contain the stimulant caffeine.*

▶ *Take regular daily exercise.*

▶ *Keep to a regular sleep schedule.*

▶ *Have a milky drink and banana, or a snack of complex carbohydrate such as rice crackers, before bedtime. This can stimulate brain chemicals that induce and maintain sleep.*

▶ *Take time to relax before bed by having a bath or reading a book or magazine.*

Your general health, diet, fitness and psychological health can all influence your susceptibility to pain and the way you perceive pain. With an understanding of your body's needs, you can improve your lifestyle and minimise pain.

### TREATING YOUR BODY RIGHT

In considering how to deal with pain, or how to minimise the potential threat of pain, it is important to think of the body and the mind as a whole and not just the parts of the body where pain occurs. The recognition that all aspects of your lifestyle such as your diet, posture, fitness and state of mind and spirit contribute to your well-being is known as the holistic approach to health. If you learn to treat yourself right according to the needs of your body, mind and spirit, pain caused by an unhealthy or unsuitable lifestyle may be avoided.

Your body is very effective at providing warning signs when you are run down: tiredness and aches and pains can all be telling you to take urgent action to change your lifestyle. Changing potentially harmful habits will prevent the development of more serious illnesses.

### Eat a balanced diet

Many painful diseases and illnesses can be directly linked to poor dietary habits. A high-fat diet, for example, is known to contribute to hypertension and heart disease. Understanding which foods are high in fat, such as crisps and mayonnaise, can help you to make responsible decisions about which foods to include in a healthy diet. A well-balanced diet of foods containing protein, carbohydrates, fibre, vitamins and minerals in the right proportions (see page 57) can greatly improve your health by raising the body's natural defence mechanisms, making you less prone to illness.

### Take regular exercise

Regular exercise can help to prevent the pain caused by certain disorders, such as angina. In general, exercising regularly will help to maintain a healthy body weight and also relieve stress, which may heighten existing pain. More specifically, exercise can reduce the risk of pain caused by heart disease by helping to reduce blood pressure and cholesterol levels.

### Get enough sleep

Regular sleep is important for you to function well and safely during the day. In the short term, sleep deprivation leads to irritability and a shortened attention span; over long periods, people find it increasingly difficult to concentrate and their energy levels deteriorate. Sleep deprivation may also lower the immune system, exposing sufferers to the risk of pain caused by low grade illnesses such as viral infections. Depression and fatigue caused by lack of sleep can also exacerbate any existing pain. Although the amount of sleep required varies between individuals, and changes with age, adults generally need between seven and eight hours sleep a night.

### Reduce your alcohol intake

Initially medical advice on alcohol intake for optimum health may seem confusing. Moderate drinking is now thought to be beneficial to health. Current recommendations are that men can consume up to four units of alcohol per day and women three, with one or two alcohol-free days per week.

A unit is defined as a small glass of wine, half a pint of beer or a single measure of spirits. Drinking too much on a regular basis can lead to mental and physical health problems. Hangovers with headaches and stomachaches are common. Long-term alcohol abuse can cause chronic inflammation of the stomach and, in more serious cases, cirrhosis of the liver. Excessive alcohol intake can also weaken the heart muscle, reducing the efficiency of its pumping action.

## Giving up smoking

Smoking may cause the development and aggravation of a range of painful diseases including asthma and bronchitis, heart disease, cancer, particularly of the lungs, and stomach problems such as ulcers, gastritis and indigestion. There is a suggestion that smoking may cause damaged tissues to take more time to heal because the nicotine contributes to the narrowing of blood vessels, thus reducing the flow of blood into the tissues to start the healing process.

Women who smoke may also be more likely to develop osteoporosis, a painful condition common in post-menopausal women causing the bones to become brittle. It is also worth remembering that non-smokers exposed to tobacco smoke have an increased risk of contracting cancer. Although stopping smoking requires great willpower, the risks of developing serious disease begin to reduce as soon as you give up.

### STEPS TO GIVING UP SMOKING

The following methods may help to bolster your determination to give up smoking:

▶ *Set a date for quitting completely. Seek out a non-smoking friend who can help you to monitor your progress.*

▶ *Write a list of the advantages of giving up. Put it in a prominent position, such as in your diary or in the kitchen so you see it often.*

▶ *Develop new interests, such as taking up a sport or a hobby.*

▶ *Make time for relaxation to reduce stress, thus reducing the urge to smoke.*

▶ *Congratulate yourself frequently on your progress.*

▶ *Save the money you would have spent on cigarettes and buy yourself regular treats, such as a new CD.*

## LOOKING AFTER YOUR BODY

By making the right choices for your body, you can help to improve your emotional and physical health and also increase your life expectancy. Take steps to adopt a healthier lifestyle by eating a well-balanced diet, exercising regularly, giving up smoking, and keeping your alcohol consumption at moderate levels.

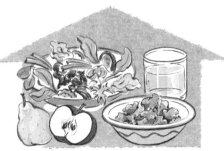

*BALANCING YOUR DIET*
*A varied diet with complex carbohydrates, protein, fibre and reduced fat together with adequate levels of vitamins and minerals can help to improve the way you look and feel.*

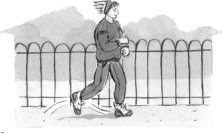

*INCREASING EXERCISE*
*Regular exercise such as jogging can help to keep the joints flexible and prevent stiffness. It also improves the blood circulation and reduces the risk of heart disease.*

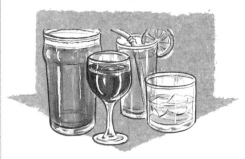

*CUTTING DOWN ON ALCOHOL*
*A safe daily maximum intake of alcohol is 4 units for men and 3 units for women (1 unit equals half a pint of beer or cider, 1 measure of spirits, or 1 small glass of wine).*

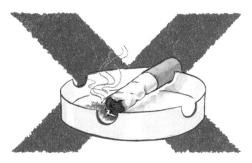

*KICKING THE SMOKING HABIT*
*Smoking is one of the major causes of avoidable disease, so it makes sense to give up. Remember, too, that passive smoking can increase the risk of lung disease.*

# MANAGING STRESS

*A certain amount of stress is good for people as it stimulates and motivates them. However, in the long term too much or inappropriate stress can lead to many painful disorders.*

When you feel that your ability to cope is being outweighed by the demands put on you, stress has reached the point where it can have a harmful effect. This kind and level of stress can cause actual physical damage to the body.

### HOW STRESS AFFECTS PAIN

Stress can be caused by external pressures, such as the demands forced upon you by family, work or study. It can also be the result of internal pressures, such as illness, pain, anxiety or depression.

During stress the brain alerts the hypothalamus, a small part of the brain that controls body functions such as temperature, sleep and appetite. The hypothalamus triggers the release of a variety of hormones which cause some typical body reactions such as raised blood pressure, a rapid heartbeat and increased breathing rate. While this may be a useful response when faced by sudden danger, excessive long-term stress can lead to serious pain problems. In the early stages, stress can cause migraine, stomachache, indigestion and nausea. It can also result in longer-term problems such as heart disease and backache. Stress can even heighten existing pain because part of the stress response is heightened sensitivity to all stimuli and increased muscle tension. For all of these reasons it's essential to examine the level of stress in your life and develop techniques to manage it more effectively.

## Identifying stress factors

The first step towards managing stress in your life is to identify specifically what makes you feel stressed. This is not necessarily as straightforward as it sounds, as signs of stress such as fatigue and depression may not always be immediately obvious. However, you should try to analyse the frequency of particular stress symptoms as they relate to specific situations in your life. Typical physical signs of stress include headaches, teethgrinding, aching shoulders, neck and back, nausea, ulcers, indigestion, diarrhoea or constipation, shortness of breath, heart palpitations, cold hands and feet, and skin problems. First try to become aware of the physical symptoms you experience when you are stressed. Then analyse when such symptoms occur in relation to the other events happening in your life. A diary may be useful for this purpose.

## Dealing with environmental stress

Your environment can contribute to the impact of stress in your daily life. The pace of modern urban life, the crowding, noise and constant change, as well as the isolation

---

### THE PAIN–STRESS CYCLE

A little stress helps to motivate, but too much can lead to a vicious spiral of stress-related illnesses, such as tension and insomnia, resulting in an increased perception of pain.

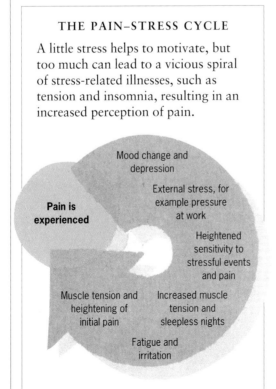

Mood change and depression

External stress, for example pressure at work

Pain is experienced

Heightened sensitivity to stressful events and pain

Muscle tension and heightening of initial pain

Increased muscle tension and sleepless nights

Fatigue and irritation

---

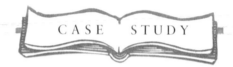
# The Headache Sufferer

*Many people suffer regular headaches – perhaps once a week or more. A common type is the tension headache, caused by stress and exacerbated by lack of exercise and a poor diet. Painkillers may provide relief initially, but they do not address the symptoms in the long term. Learning to relax and improving your overall health can reduce or even eliminate these headaches.*

John, a 31-year-old advertising executive, has suffered headaches for years, but since his promotion six months ago they have increased in frequency and intensity, and are now occurring almost daily. The pain feels like a band of pressure around the head and down the neck. John has been taking painkillers but these are not really helping anymore.

John's doctor diagnoses that he is suffering from tension headaches caused by stress and exacerbated by excessive drinking and smoking, poor diet and lack of exercise. The doctor advises him to cut down on painkillers, to learn relaxation exercises, and to limit or give up drinking and smoking. He also advises John to improve his diet and take up regular exercise.

## WHAT SHOULD JOHN DO?

John should learn to do simple relaxation exercises, such as deep breathing, which can be done at work or at home and take only a few minutes. Relaxation books and tapes can also be helpful. In addition, he should stop smoking, cut down on alcohol and junk food, and start eating meals with high nutritional value.

He should introduce some exercise into his daily routine. Short, daily walks will improve circulation and reduce muscle tension.

Finally, John should try to ease pressure at work, for example, by delegating work to other staff, by organising his schedule more carefully and by not taking on more than he can handle.

## Action Plan

**WORK**
*Delegate work to junior staff. Reorganise schedules, allowing time for a one-week holiday.*

**EXERCISE**
*Walk for half an hour every day and swim once a week. At work, get up from the desk regularly and move around.*

**LIFESTYLE**
*Start taking healthy lunches to work. Start a programme to stop smoking and reduce alcohol to a maximum of two drinks per day. Learn relaxation exercises and practise at least twice daily.*

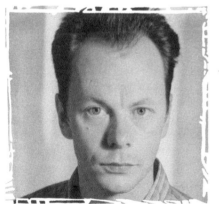

**WORK**
*Pressure at work to meet tight deadlines and employer's expectations can cause tension headaches.*

**EXERCISE**
*Lack of exercise can contribute to high stress levels increasing the risk of suffering from tension headaches.*

**LIFESTYLE**
*Fast food, cigarettes, alcohol and a lack of sleep reduce the body's ability to deal with stress.*

## HOW THINGS TURNED OUT FOR JOHN

John eased the pressure at work by rescheduling some deadlines. He has started to go for a 30-minute walk every morning and practises deep breathing exercises at work. He has cut down on smoking and alcohol and doesn't rely on fast food so much. An aromatherapy masseur showed him how to do self-massage on his neck and shoulders to ease the tension. Overall, his headaches have eased and he feels much healthier generally.

## Relieving stress with counselling

Many people find professional counselling can help them to cope with chronic stress symptoms. Counselling can take many forms, from assertiveness training to assist you to express your needs more effectively, to more personal psychotherapy which may assist in the treatment of more deeply rooted causes of stress, such as emotional problems, poor self-esteem, anxiety and depression.

# STEPS TO COPING WITH STRESS

Recognising and reducing harmful stress is one of the most important steps you can take to minimise or circumvent episodes of certain stress-related pain. It isn't possible or even desirable to avoid the challenge of stress in life, but there are steps you can take to help you cope when stress gets out of hand.

▶ *Eat a balanced diet. An inadequate diet will deplete your body of the resources it needs to deal with life's demands.*

▶ *Ensure you get adequate sleep. Sleep deprivation can cause stress, which in turn can cause insomnia.*

▶ *Exercise regularly. Physical exercise helps to relieve tension, and to build up your general health, making you more resistant to illness and disease.*

▶ *Learn to relax. Make time for walking or gardening. You may find it easier to learn to relax by practising techniques such as meditation or yoga in a group.*

▶ *Practise visualisation techniques. Imagining yourself in a pleasant setting can help promote feelings of relaxation. Visualising a positive outcome to the problem that is causing stress can also help to reduce stress-related symptoms.*

▶ *Think positively. Try to look at experiences that induce feelings of anger and depression in a positive way.*

many people feel, can all create stress. A common theme in environmental stress is a feeling of loss of control, a sense that the individual is powerless.

It is important to regain a sense of control over your environment. Assess the daily activities that cause you stress and consider how to avoid or alleviate them. For example, if driving a car in heavy traffic makes you tense and anxious, explore public transport options. If external noise is an irritant in your home environment, look at the possibility of double glazing your windows, hanging heavy curtains, or even blocking external noise by playing background tapes. Recordings of sounds such as waves or instrumental music can be very soothing.

## Coping with stress in relationships

Stress is often caused by day-to-day communication and personal relationships. Family relationships can be put at risk by demands from children and other family members. For example, younger children may have difficulty sleeping at night which can exhaust parents, while older children may resent their lack of freedom and sulk causing the parents to feel additional stress.

Stress can also be caused by placing excessive demands on yourself. For example, a manager starting a new job may become stressed by trying to impress her colleagues, and by trying to meet their expectations. Trying to emulate those who appear more successful than oneself can lead to feelings of inadequacy, which can also cause stress.

When personal relationships are affected many people suppress their emotion instead of communicating directly. This can lead to physically painful symptoms as feelings of anger, frustration, or distress, if not allowed direct and constructive expression, can frequently manifest themselves in physical symptoms such as headaches, nervous tics, palpitations and hyperventilation.

Communication is the first step towards overcoming stress in personal relationships. In the long term it is one of the most effective ways of alleviating stress and bringing about constructive change in your life.

# ENCOURAGING POSITIVE THINKING

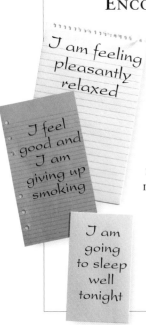

J am feeling pleasantly relaxed

J feel good and J am giving up smoking

J am going to sleep well tonight

One way to encourage positive thinking is to bombard your mind with positive thought intentions. For example, telling yourself 'I feel good and I am giving up smoking', is far more positive than the negative 'I am not going to smoke any more'. You can reinforce the message by writing out positive thoughts and placing them at eye level around the workplace and home. If you have made a conscious decision not to get tense during the day, put up positive messages such as 'I am feeling pleasantly relaxed', and 'I am going to sleep well tonight'. Repeating these positive phrases to yourself even when stressed, helps to replace negative 'what's the use?' self sabotage thoughts. Thinking positively may help to counteract a pain problem before it escalates.

# FOOD AGAINST PAIN

*Many types of pain can be prevented by a healthy diet rich in essential nutrients. Once these have become a way of life, your body should become less susceptible to painful health problems.*

A poor diet can contribute to many painful conditions. The pain caused by heart disease, stroke, stomach ulcers, osteoporosis, shingles, migraine and certain cancers can often be alleviated or avoided altogether by eating the right foods in the right amounts.

### EATING WELL TO FEEL GOOD
A well-balanced diet containing protein, complex carbohydrates, minerals, vitamins and fibre is essential for maintaining the body's natural mechanisms. For example, if you don't have enough fibre in your diet, you may suffer pain from constipation. Too much saturated fat in your diet can aggravate or even bring on painful heart ailments such as angina. Many stomach complaints are caused by eating too many rich foods. Too much sugar can cause tooth decay. Eating certain kinds of food can also make

a significant difference to the management of a particular painful illness. For example evidence has now shown that polyunsaturated fats found in fish oils can have an anti-inflammatory effect on the joints of some arthritis sufferers. You can help to counteract arthritis and many other painful disorders by decreasing the amount of problem foods such as animal fats.

## Vitamins and minerals
Eating a variety of fruit and vegetables is important because they contain vitamins and minerals. Although your body only needs small quantities of these nutrients, they play an important part in protecting you from pain caused by illness and disease.

A lack of vitamins and minerals in your diet can lead to specific illnesses and pain. For example, a deficiency of $B_1$ can cause fatigue, muscle weakness and nausea, while

## CAPSULE FOR HEALTH

One of the best ways of promoting good health is to eat a balanced diet. This should contain a healthy balance of complex carbohydrates such as vegetables, cereals and fruit; protein from meat, fish, nuts, eggs and pulses; and fat from vegetable oil, seeds, nuts,

oily fish and dairy products. Nutritionists agree that generally we should eat more complex carbohydrates and eat less saturated fat. This is found primarily in dairy products and red meat. Saturated fats can clog the arteries and contribute to heart disease and stroke.

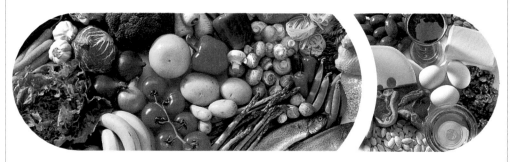

**For a healthy diet** eat these foods in abundance; the products on the right should be eaten in moderation.

## FIGHTING PAIN WITH VITAMINS AND MINERALS

A healthy, balanced diet includes sufficient amounts of all the vitamins and minerals. Studies show that chronic pain sufferers are often deficient in some vitamins and minerals as the stress of pain can deplete these nutrients in the body. The table below shows the main sources of these nutrients and the recommended daily allowance (RDA). If taking supplements without specialist advice take care not to exceed the RDA over a long period.

| NUTRIENT | SOURCES | RDA: MEN | RDA: WOMEN | FUNCTION |
|---|---|---|---|---|
| Vitamin B$_1$ | Wholemeal bread, cereals, pulses, nuts, potatoes, pork, liver, heart, kidneys | 1.0 mg | 0.8 mg | B complex vitamins play a vital part in most processes in the body including manufacture of red blood cells and release of energy from food. They are essential for healthy skin and correct functioning of brain and nervous system. They may help to prevent the onset of nerve pain, and relieve period pain and depression. Women need to take folic acid supplements (400 mcg) before conception and during early pregnancy to avoid neural tube defects, such as spina bifida, in the developing foetus. |
| Vitamin B$_2$ | Cereals, dairy foods, meat, fish, poultry, eggs | 1.3 mg | 1.1 mg | |
| Vitamin B$_3$ | Rice, pulses, meat, fish, eggs | 17 mg | 13 mg | |
| Vitamin B$_6$ | Wholemeal bread, nuts, soya, bananas poultry, meat, fish, eggs | 1.4 mg | 1.2 mg | |
| Vitamin B$_{12}$ | Cereals, dairy foods, meat, fish, eggs | 1.5 mcg | 1.5 mcg | |
| Folic acid | Wholemeal bread, cereals, nuts, pulses, green leafy vegetables, liver | 200 mcg | 200 mcg | |
| Vitamin C | Citrus fruit, blackcurrants, kiwi fruit, fresh vegetables, potatoes | 40 mg | 40 mg | Antioxidant; leads to healthy teeth and gums; promotes healing of wounds. |
| Vitamin D | Dairy foods, oily fish, margarine, eggs (Also from action of sunlight on skin) | 10 mcg | 10 mcg | Heals bones; can prevent osteoporosis and osteoarthritis. |
| Vitamin E | Wheatgerm, cereals, nuts, seeds, vegetable oils, sweet potato | 4 mg minimum* | 3 mg minimum* | Antioxidant; may relieve breast pain and leg cramps; may help prevent heart disease. |
| Calcium | Wholemeal cereals, sesame seeds, green leafy vegetables, dairy foods, oily fish, | 700 mg | 700 mg | Muscle and nerve function; healthy bones and teeth; can prevent osteoporosis, osteoarthritis. |

*Higher doses of Vitamin E may help reduce the risk of cancer and heart disease. Extra Vitamin E is often recommended for those recovering from heart attack*

a deficiency of vitamin B$_2$ can cause dry and cracked skin and sore lips and tongue. Calcium deficiency can lead to back pain and susceptibility to fractures. The table above shows the function of a number of vitamins and minerals. Vitamins can also help in pain recovery. For example, vitamin C can help promote wound healing and fight recurrent infections. It may also promote sleep as it helps produce serotonin, a neurotransmitter that helps calm the mind.

### Food allergies and intolerances

Some types of pain, such as migraine, headache and abdominal pain, may be triggered by eating particular kinds of foods. The most common trigger foods include cereals, dairy products, caffeine-based products, yeast-based items, shellfish and citrus fruits. You may be allergic to one or other of these foods, or, more commonly, you may have a food intolerance. A food allergy is an abnormal response by the immune system to an otherwise harmless food substance. A food intolerance is also an adverse reaction to something in the diet, but it does not involve the immune system. For example, the body may lack an enzyme needed to digest a particular dietary substance. Sufferers from coeliac disease have an intolerance to gluten found in wheat and other cereals. The condition damages the lining of the intestine so that essential nutrients cannot properly be absorbed into the body.

Both conditions cause a range of symptoms including headaches and indigestion, as well as chronic illnesses such as eczema and irritable bowel syndrome. The cause of a food allergy or intolerance is found by eliminating suspect foods from the diet, then reintroducing them one at a time while watching for adverse reactions. Such investigations should not be undertaken without the supervision of a doctor or nutritionist.

# EXERCISE AS PAIN PREVENTION

*Exercise is vital for good health, helping to keep the body flexible and improve the circulation. By keeping active you can help to prevent painful illnesses and disease.*

When suffering pain, the body's natural instinct is to rest and minimise activity. If you are suffering from an acute pain condition, such as severe joint inflammation, rest is generally advised because movement can aggravate existing damage. Likewise, if you are experiencing chronic pain, you may find it difficult to incorporate exercise into your life.

However, as soon as possible exercise should be reintroduced, as prolonged inactivity can be very harmful to your general well-being. Unused muscles contract and become weak, and are more likely to go into painful spasm. Arthritis sufferers, in particular, need to keep their joints as mobile and flexible as possible. Lack of exercise in general can make you feel weak, fatigued and breathless, and your circulation will be adversely affected. Inactivity over a long period can lead to bone damage and weakening of muscles which make recovery from illness far more difficult.

In addition, exercise can stimulate the production of endorphins, the body's natural painkiller. Lack of exercise leads to low levels of endorphins in the bloodstream, in turn increasing the body's susceptibility to pain and compounding the problem by increasing the risk of psychological disorders, such as depression.

## What kind of exercise and how much?

There is a wide range of exercise options available. In the first instance you should consult your doctor or a physiotherapist as to how much and what kind of exercise to take to help alleviate your particular pain problem. For example, if you have a painful back or stiff joints that may become more stressed by weight-bearing exercises, non-weight bearing exercise, such as swimming, may be helpful. On the other hand, if you are suffering from osteoporosis, weight-bearing exercises may be what you need as they strengthen bones. It is also useful to think about non-conventional forms of exercise. T'ai chi (see page 75) and yoga (see page 74), for example, can be very beneficial for back, neck and shoulder pain. Both forms of exercise strengthen muscles, improve posture and can aid relaxation.

Most experts agree that the ideal level of activity for adults is 20 to 30 minutes of exercise that raises the pulse and respiration, at least three times a week, but preferably every day. Obviously the extent to which you are able to exercise will depend on the amount of pain experienced, but even small amounts of activity on a daily basis can make an enormous difference.

## Going to a gym

Specific machines in your local gym can be very useful for strengthening muscles and joints affected by specific pain problems. If attending a gym for the first time, ask your doctor for a checkup before you go.

At your first session you will probably be asked about your current state of health and medical history. It is important to tell the instructor if you are taking any medication and if you have a medical condition or disability. The instructor will then work out an exercise programme for you which will be closely monitored and reviewed. The instructor will also teach you about the benefits of the various exercise machines and how to use them, and also whether they are suitable for your needs and state of health. Your exercise programme will ensure that the intensity and the time you spend on a machine will both build up gradually.

*EXERCISING SAFELY*
*Exercise machines can be dangerous and should be used with caution. Always consult a trainer before use.*

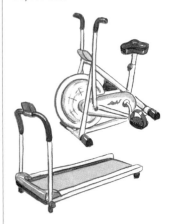

**Exercise bicycles and treadmills** can be adjusted to your fitness level. Increase the level of difficulty as you improve.

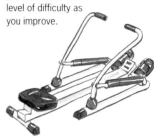

**Rowing machines** provide an all-round work-out. If you have back, knee, shoulder or neck pain, check with a doctor first.

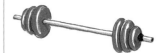

**Weightlifting** is a great body strengthener and toner. Ask a trainer to explain the different types of weights before use.

## Stretches for a
# Sedentary Lifestyle

*Sitting in a chair, whether a car seat, armchair or desk chair, for long periods, particularly with poor posture, puts pressure on the spinal discs, so that they flatten and lose their cushioning action. This makes the back vulnerable to chronic pain.*

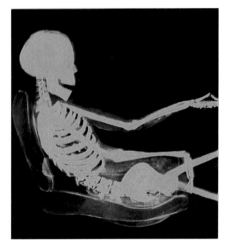

**COUCH POTATO**
*Slumping on the sofa can do great damage to your back. Gradually it may become more curved and the lack of support may cause your muscles to tense.*

Sedentary lifestyles have become an increasing feature of modern society. Up to 14 hours a day may be spent seated – at home, at work, in the car or on a train. Such prolonged sitting can easily tire the back and make it vulnerable to back problems when over-stretching or twisting. When sitting in the same position for a long period, the back muscles become stretched. In particular, slumping in a chair without good back support increases the risk of cramp and pain in the lower and mid back areas, and the neck and shoulders.

Driving for extended periods can exacerbate the problem as the back muscles become tense and strained when going around corners and accelerating. In addition, bumps in the road can jolt the spine and cause bruising of the joints.

**Action plan** Try to change position frequently and get up to do tasks, rather than sitting still for long periods. If a long journey is necessary, plan regular short stops where you can walk around. Some simple exercises may relieve the pressure, stretch the spine and improve posture. These can be done in your chair or standing up. Always do exercises gently and stop immediately if they cause any pain.

## CHAIR EXERCISES

There are several exercises you can do without leaving your chair. They will help you to stretch your back, and also relieve tension and stress. Prepare by sitting up with your neck and shoulders relaxed, feet flat on the ground and hands in your lap.

**1** *Concentrate on your breathing while slowly rolling your head. Shrug your shoulders when finished.*

**Roll your head** down and up, and then to the left and right

**2** *Keep back and neck straight and clasp your hands behind the chair. Raise them a little way and look up.*

**Be careful** not to strain your muscles

**Pull in your stomach** and 'sit tall'

**3** *With palms facing outward, raise your arms above your head, breathing in at the same time, and clasp hands. Hold for a count of five.*

## Avoiding injury when exercising

For those who haven't exercised for a long time, whether through choice or through immobility due to injury or illness, it is essential to seek your doctor's advice before beginning any exercise regime and to build up a routine gradually.

If you have decided to start a new exercise programme, remember to wear loose, comfortable clothes such as a tracksuit or lightweight cotton shorts with an aerated cotton top or shirt that will allow the body to breathe. Women should make sure that they are wearing a well-fitting support bra. For active sports, use sturdy, non-slip trainers with cushioned soles which will reduce jarring of the knees, hips and spine. They are also essential when jogging.

All exercise and sport routines require warming up and cooling down exercises (see page 27). Warming up before exercise helps to prevent joint and muscle injuries, while cooling down afterwards brings the heart rate back down gently.

If your joints are stiff in the morning you can help to relieve the stiffness by having a warm bath or shower first before taking exercise. After your bath or shower you can relax stiff or sore joints by gently extending and flexing the joints as far as they can comfortably stretch. Lightly massaging painful joints and the back and neck areas with warmed olive oil can also help to improve your flexibility and enhance the blood circulation through the muscles, thus helping to prevent muscle spasm.

## EXERCISING AND YOUR LIFESTYLE

Regular exercise brings greater benefits than infrequent bouts of physical activity. Daily exercise performed without a break for just 12 minutes will make the body fitter by improving the efficiency of the heart and lungs. To build up a routine, try exercising at the same time each day, working up to 30 minutes or more per session. Choose a form of exercise that fits easily into your current lifestyle. It could be as simple as taking a brisk walk to your local shops for small items rather than driving or relying on home delivery.

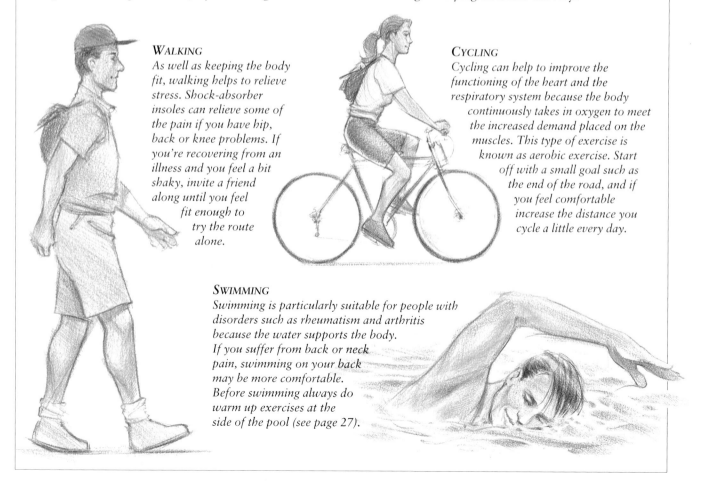

### WALKING
As well as keeping the body fit, walking helps to relieve stress. Shock-absorber insoles can relieve some of the pain if you have hip, back or knee problems. If you're recovering from an illness and you feel a bit shaky, invite a friend along until you feel fit enough to try the route alone.

### CYCLING
Cycling can help to improve the functioning of the heart and the respiratory system because the body continuously takes in oxygen to meet the increased demand placed on the muscles. This type of exercise is known as aerobic exercise. Start off with a small goal such as the end of the road, and if you feel comfortable increase the distance you cycle a little every day.

### SWIMMING
Swimming is particularly suitable for people with disorders such as rheumatism and arthritis because the water supports the body. If you suffer from back or neck pain, swimming on your back may be more comfortable. Before swimming always do warm up exercises at the side of the pool (see page 27).

# CORRECT POSTURE

*Many serious aches and pains result from poor posture. By improving your posture, you may be able to prevent severe and possibly long-term back and neck pains from developing.*

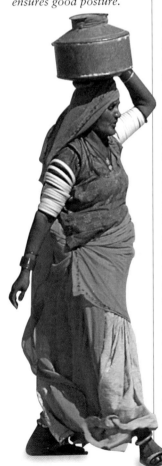

Look at any healthy baby or toddler sitting on the floor and you will see that their back posture is beautifully straight. Unfortunately, however, most people's posture deteriorates as they age. With our increasingly sedentary lifestyle, people can sit for hours at a time – often in poor seating – in the car, at home, in schools and colleges and in the workplace. Over the years bad posture can lead to loss of muscle tone and ultimately severe back and neck pains, forcing sufferers to seek remedy from physical therapists.

## WHY GOOD POSTURE IS IMPORTANT

The human skeleton is covered with an interlinking system of muscles, which are connected to the bones by tendons. These act to lever and mobilise the body, and to protect the inner organs. The ligaments provide extra support. The trunk is held up by a complex layering and interweaving of back and abdominal muscles which act as a sort of natural elastic corset when toned.

However, this complicated system is easily damaged and any slight distortion of the posture can lead to limb or trunk stress and injury over time. This explains why ballet dancers, gymnasts, martial arts enthusiasts, and others who rely on having a fit body for their work, recognise the importance of good posture and work hard to build up strong trunk muscles.

Slouching or standing in awkward positions can put undue pressure on the muscles. The tendons and ligaments then have to compensate and work harder to support you, and you may start to feel an ache perhaps in the back or neck, which in turn may lead to a headache. If bad posture is not corrected, over a long period of time these general aches can turn into acute muscle pain or even a slipped disc.

By consciously adopting a better posture, for example by making an effort to sit without slouching, you can avoid incapacitating neck and back pain in the future.

Poor posture can also restrict the lungs and breathing capacity. The body needs a plentiful intake of oxygen in order to feel fresh and alert, but if the shoulders are hunched breathing may become restricted, with the result that insufficient oxygen is taken in. Good posture encourages a relaxed diaphragm which aids breathing.

### Factors affecting your posture

Good posture has long been considered to promote a healthy body. Slouching, sitting and standing up badly, and walking stiffly are all recognised as potential causes of painful muscular problems.

Your posture can also be affected by your weight. For the body to work and move well, it is essential to maintain a reasonable and adequate weight for your height. If you are overweight you may experience problems carrying around the extra weight as your joints will be under greater strain. Being too thin causes different problems: your body may simply lack the stamina and strength to function effectively.

Injury and pain can also affect your posture. People with advanced rheumatoid arthritis, or with osteoporosis, for example,

> ### CAUTION
> *If you have had recent surgery, a spinal or neck injury, a heart or thyroid problem, hypertension, a past severe head injury, if you are a diabetic, take sedatives or steroids or if you feel dizzy, check with your doctor before beginning a posture correction programme.*

## *Preventing Back Pain with*

# Improved Posture

*Learning to walk, sit and stand with the correct posture can be enormously beneficial for both the relief and prevention of back pain. Good posture can also help you to avoid injury when bending over or lifting.*

Poor posture can be a cause of back pain in itself. It can also exacerbate damage from other causes and lead to problems in other areas of the body. Before you can start to improve your posture, you need to assess the way you hold and move your body. The 'wall test' (see right) can help to establish a natural, comfortable posture that allows you to move and stand with a minimum of distortion and stress. Practise this for a minute or two every day, and try visualising standing and walking with a relaxed posture to help you to focus on the correct stance.

Lifting is said to be the most common cause of back pain. The damage usually occurs when people lift without thinking or when they are under pressure. When people are in a hurry, they are more likely to twist when bending down or lifting and this puts the back at maximum risk. Always assess the situation before picking something up. Is it too heavy? Do you need help? When you do lift something, make sure that you stoop and lift in the correct fashion (see below), supporting the weight with your legs so that you protect the spine from damage.

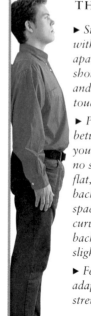

### THE WALL TEST

▶ *Stand against a wall with your feet slightly apart. Your head, shoulders, buttocks and heels should touch the wall.*

▶ *Place one hand flat between the wall and your back. If there is no space you have a flat, possibly tight back. If there is lots of space your back is too curved. Ideally your back should be just slightly curved.*

▶ *Feel how you should adapt your posture to strengthen your back.*

## LIFTING

When bending to lift things breathe out and bend the knees. Keep the back straight and move slowly and carefully. Never flex the spine while bent over. Stand up slowly, holding your abdomen in to act as a corset. Keep the object close to your chest.

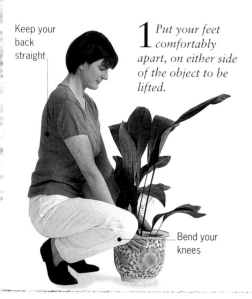

Keep your back straight

**1** *Put your feet comfortably apart, on either side of the object to be lifted.*

Bend your knees

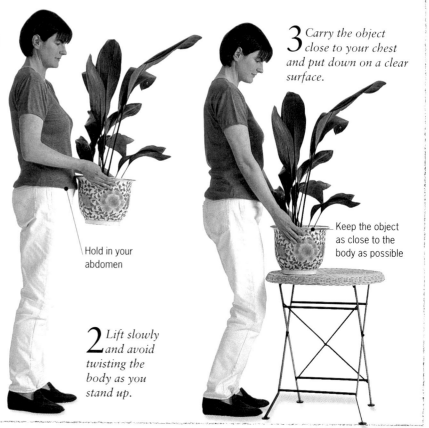

Hold in your abdomen

**2** *Lift slowly and avoid twisting the body as you stand up.*

**3** *Carry the object close to your chest and put down on a clear surface.*

Keep the object as close to the body as possible

## BUYING A BED

Spend time choosing the right bed to avoid such problems as chronic back pain. The following points are worth bearing in mind:

▶ *Make sure the mattress is comfortable but provides firm support. Buy a good quality one that will not sag with use (see below).*

▶ *Take into account your sleeping habits when choosing a bed – you take up more room if you sleep on your side, for example – and buy the widest you can afford.*

▶ *If buying a double bed, make sure both you and your partner try it first.*

▶ *Make sure the bed is at least 15 cm (6 in) longer than you or your partner – whoever is taller.*

▶ *If there is a big weight difference between you and your partner, consider a pocket-spring mattress or twin beds – otherwise you will keep rolling together in your sleep.*

will find that their posture becomes distorted through no fault of their own. If you suffer from stress, you may find that your head, stomach and back become tensed, causing pain. In response you'll find that you tense your body against the pain which over time can lead to general stiffness and distortion. Adopting a better posture can also help to relax cramped muscles.

Wearing comfortable shoes can make all the difference to freedom of movement and your body alignment when walking or running. High heels tip the pelvis forward and over-arch the back, affecting balance and causing an unnatural stance which places strain on the back, knees and feet.

Your clothes can also influence the way you move. Tight clothes or heavy outdoor winter-wear can weigh the shoulders down, limit breathing capacity and affect movement. Loose, light clothes are the least restricting to free movement. Even the weather can affect your body posture: cold and windy weather can cause you to tense and tighten your muscles and squash the lungs by holding the body in to keep warm.

### Adopting a good posture

Posture is developed without conscious thought from an early age. People rarely think about their posture unless the body begins to ache for one reason or another. Demonstrating how best to move, sit and stand with a relaxed, aware and stress-free musculature is far more complex. One of

the greatest difficulties in adopting better posture is in correcting entrenched physical misalignments. However, it's worth persevering to change bad habits.

You can take steps to help your body naturally into a better physical alignment. Always try to walk with your back straight, pulling your shoulders back, keeping your stomach in and lifting your chest and ribs. Whether walking, standing or sitting it may help to picture a string attached to the centre of the top of the head. Imagine that this string gently pulls the body up with every slight movement you make by pulling your shoulders back, lifting your chest and realigning the body.

Regular stretching and muscle strengthening exercises may help to prevent severe back or neck pain and tension headaches. Many injuries are caused by sudden movement after a period of inactivity. For example, lifting heavy items after sitting all day in a low chair can lead to back problems. Always warm up muscles sufficiently before any vigorous movement (see page 27).

A healthy posture relies upon a relaxed mind and body interplay. An angry or aggressive person has a totally different posture from someone who is laughing and happy. You can promote a more relaxed posture by decreasing your stress levels and reducing the tension in your life.

### SLEEP AND POSTURE

Bad sleeping positions can cause severe chronic back and neck pain. You may think that the position in which you sleep is beyond your control, yet there are a number of changes you can make to prevent or ease pain.

### Choosing the right bed

The first step towards achieving a good sleeping posture is to get rid of your old mattress when it no longer provides adequate support and to buy a suitable new one (see left). Sagging mattresses can cause or make back pain worse, and you may wake up stiff and sore.

Waterbeds can provide firm support to the body and are often used in hospitals for patients with painful joints and limbs or bedsores. Japanese futon mattresses have become popular and are said to be effective for backache. However, they may be too hard for those with chronic back pain.

## SELECTING THE IDEAL MATTRESS

A medium-firm to firm – but not too hard – bed is essential as it allows the spine to relax and re-lengthen during sleep.

It's best to put your mattress on a slatted base or a spring base so that moisture doesn't get trapped in the mattress.

*NIGHT SUPPORT*
*A pocket-spring mattress gives excellent support to the whole body, as each spring moves independently to support the body. A spring base must be used with this kind of bed.*

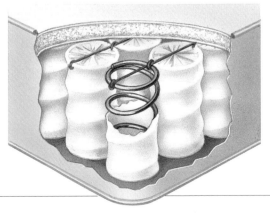

# IMPROVING YOUR SLEEPING POSTURE

As roughly a third of your life is spent in bed, it is essential that you have a good sleeping posture. A bad sleeping position can lead to chronic back and neck pain. The following suggestions may help people who already suffer such pain.

**Supporting the neck**
Specially contoured pillows are available which give extra support to the neck. These pillows help to 'cushion' the neck if it hurts to turn over in bed.

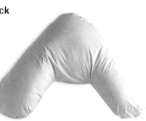

**Improvising at home**
If you find your pillow doesn't cushion your neck enough try tying a ribbon round the middle of your pillow.

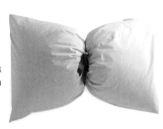

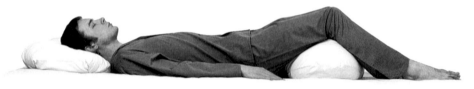

*SUPPORTING THE BACK*
*If sleeping on your back, you can avoid straining your lower back by lying with your* knees bent so your feet are flat on the bed. You may find it more comfortable to slip a soft pillow under the knees for support.

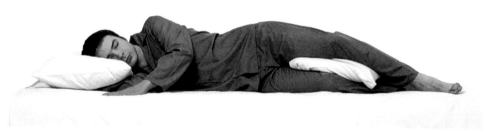

*SUPPORTING THE KNEES AND HIPS*
*If you have aching hips or knees or a painful back placing a pillow or cushion between the* knees or thighs may help you to sleep on your side. This position eases the pain as it stops the pelvis pulling on the lower back.

If you are sleeping with a partner, the mattress may start to dip in the middle and this can cause back pain. With a good bed base you should not have a problem but if it does occur, or if you and your partner prefer different types of mattresses, you may find that twin beds or a split mattress provides the answer.

## Adopting a good sleeping posture
To relax the body and promote a comfortable sleeping position, try breathing exercises before sleeping. Breathe in and out calmly and slowly to reduce tension in the back. Imagine that you can really feel your back letting go of any pain and tension. Visualise any pain draining away from your back, and you should feel more and more at ease. Gently wriggle your feet and toes and stretch both legs to aid circulation and to prevent stiffness.

If you suffer from chronic back pain, you may find it uncomfortable to lie on your back. However, by keeping your knees bent with your feet flat on the bed you can prevent additional strain and pull to the lower back when lying down.

Turning over in bed can present major problems for back pain sufferers. A wide, purpose-made, soft fabric belt with a velcro fastening offers extra support for the back when turning over or getting out of bed.

## HELPING CHILDREN TO DEVELOP GOOD POSTURE

Encouraging schoolchildren to stand and sit straight is not just a matter of basic discipline. Sitting and standing up straight are important factors in avoiding back and neck pain later in life.

▶ *Make sure that your child's school bag is not too heavy. Check that the shoulders are relaxed and balanced when carrying the bag so that there is no strain on the back.*

▶ *If your child has a paper round, suggest that he or she wheels a bike supporting the heavy newspaper bag.*

▶ *Watch your child's weight – being overweight can affect your child's posture.*

▶ *Check that your child's desk and chair are an appropriate size and are not leading to bad postural habits.*

▶ *Make sure that your child's school desk and chair are appropriate – all school furniture should be examined regularly from a health and safety perspective.*

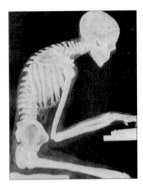

**BAD HABITS**
*Bad posture at the computer can cause a variety of aches and pains, such as back pain, eye strain and wrist complaints.*

**Seeking advice from an ergonomist**
An employer can seek advice from a health and safety ergonomist to ensure that employees are sitting correctly. An ergonomist studies individuals at work – particularly with regard to anatomical, social, biomechanical and psychological factors – and gives advice on how work practices can be made as safe, healthy and efficient as possible.

# RELAXING IN THE OFFICE

Stress in the work place can affect your posture. If you sit with tensed hunched shoulders, you can cause aches and pains in the neck and back. It is therefore important that you deal with workplace stresses and irritations and solve them as quickly and effectively as possible. There are various ways to counteract stress and tension in the office which you can put into practice immediately. If everyone in the office arena makes exercise an integral part of their daily routine it will be easier to remain motivated.

## Getting out of bed
Getting up from a horizontal position can put great strain on the back. You can prepare yourself for this potentially painful movement by doing some relaxing breathing before starting to get up. Then turn onto your side, bring both legs over the side of the bed, and raise yourself slowly into the sitting position. At this point it's a good idea to have a short rest. Then lean very slightly forward and, breathing in, try to relax your back and neck as you stand up, letting your feet and thighs take the weight. You may find that repeating a simple phrase such as 'Neck and back be free' to yourself helps to remind you that the back and neck needs to be as flexible as possible as you stand up and walk.

### OFFICE POSTURE
Many people who sit at a desk all day suffer from chronic back or neck pain. Employers are required by law to provide chairs that are of the correct height and position for each employee in relation to their desks. The tasks to be performed should also be taken into account, such as whether a computer will be used. Office chairs should therefore be adjustable so that each person is able to feel comfortable. Anyone working for long periods at a computer terminal should take regular breaks both to relax muscles and relieve eye strain.

Doing repeated tasks during the day such as typing on a computer keyboard can cause physical damage known as repetitive strain injury. In many cases correct posture can help to reduce or avoid injuries caused by repetitive movements.

► *Learn breathing exercises to help to relax.*

► *Imagine a string from the top of your head, pulling your body up into correct alignment.*

► *Take a break from your work every hour: march up and down on the spot, or do stretching exercises.*

► *Use your lunch break to take some exercise: go swimming, take a walk, or enjoy a relaxing therapy such as aromatherapy massage.*

► *Be more tolerant of your mistakes and counteract perfectionist tendencies with humour.*

## Adopting good posture in the office
The desk should be placed about elbow height when sitting upright with the arms hanging down. The office chair should have five legs on castors. The seat should be 25–30 cm (10–12 in) from the under surface of the desk. It should have a comfortably padded seat that supports the trunk and head. The lumbar support seat-back should be adjustable. A head rest support is helpful for rest periods. You should sit square to the desk, with an adjustable angled foot rest, or with the feet placed flat on the floor during typing or writing.

## Your posture at the computer
Much office work now involves the use of a computer. To avoid potential problems such as back pain and eye strain, make sure that your computer is adjusted properly.

To prevent eye strain (which can cause painful headaches) adjust the screen so that the top of the screen is at or just below eye-level. A special screen filter can reduce glare and lessen eye strain. Altering your visual point of focus at least every 20 minutes can also reduce the risk of damaging your eyes.

Wrist and arm strain can arise from rapid, tense or jerky movements if the wrists and hands are wrongly positioned. When typing, keep the arms horizontal to the desk with hands and wrists level; a wrist rest may also help. Shaking your arms and stretching your back and legs every half hour will help to relax your muscles and avoid repetitive strain injury. If you find it difficult to remember to break off work, place a small timer by your desk to remind you to take a break and adjust your posture.

CHAPTER 4

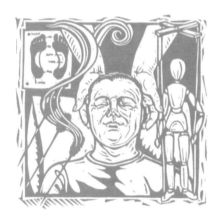

# THERAPIES FOR DEALING WITH PAIN

---

*The quest for effective pain relief has given rise to a variety of innovative techniques and approaches. Therapists have experimented with natural resources such as plants, water, heat, cold and light, and with basic tools such as hands, sticks and stones. Over time these have been refined to form a sophisticated range of natural therapies which are regularly used today to assist in the management of pain.*

---

# MIND AND BODY APPROACH

*The experience of pain is so closely involved with the brain and nervous system that the mind can play a powerful role in your effort to find effective pain relief from chronic disorders.*

Many natural healing methods use the close connection between the body, mind, vitality and spirit as the basis of their approach to pain. Some techniques use physical stimulation which eases pain in muscles and joints as well as bringing about wider physiological effects. For example, Pilates body therapy (see page 77) relieves pain by gentle stimulation and also encourages the brain to learn new patterns of muscle use so that pain is avoided in the future. Other techniques work on the principle that the mind can influence responses in the body which assist healing or relieve pain. Relaxation therapies, for instance, have been shown to relieve pain by reducing stress and relaxing the muscles.

*STRESS RELIEF*
*Many people find that painful conditions are easier to cope with if they can reduce their level of everyday stress. Activities such as gardening that provide gentle, absorbing exercise have proven beneficial for easing tension and lifting the spirits.*

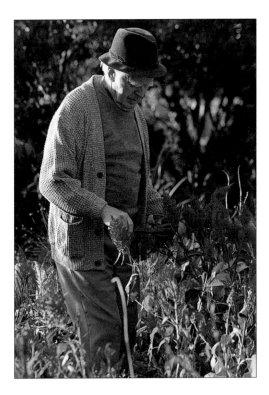

## PHYSICAL MEDICINE
Some techniques bring about physiological and energy changes in the body by using physical stimulation. For example, aromatherapy massage can relax muscles and also stimulate the release of endorphins, the body's natural painkillers. This may be one explanation behind the benefits of energy therapies such as acupuncture and shiatsu, which are said to work by acting on energy pathways in the body.

There are some methods of healing for which no physiological explanation can be given, although it is assumed that a form of energy may be involved. In therapeutic touch (see page 84), a treatment developed by Dolores Krieger, the hands of the practitioner move gently above the surface of the patient's body without actual physical contact, yet patients undergoing this treatment have claimed positive pain relief.

### Exercise
Generally, all practitioners agree that if movement is painful, especially for muscle and joint pains, you should rest. Pain is a warning signal that should not be ignored. However, there are situations where movement is beneficial. For example, arthritis sufferers need to exercise painful joints so that their movement does not become further restricted. In addition, some quite rigorous exercise programmes have been developed to treat chronic back pain. The principle behind them is that strength and flexibility are prerequisites for a stable, pain-free back.

Many osteopaths and chiropractors recommend exercises to maintain flexibility of the neck and back, once any vertebral restrictions have been attended to. Their

## CHOOSING A TREATMENT

Many painful disorders, especially chronic conditions, may be alleviated by one or more types of complementary treatment. Because stress tends to make the experience of most types of pain worse, all pain conditions can benefit from relaxation or mind control such as visualisation or meditation, and these can be used in conjunction with other pain management techniques. Before you undertake any physical treatments it is important to discuss your intentions with your doctor. She or he can advise you about any possible interactions with conventional drug treatment (as can occur with herbal medicine) and can monitor any physical changes resulting from manipulation or massage.

exercises are often based on 'muscle energy' techniques which emphasise 'stretching the strong to strengthen the weak'. In other words, rather than trying to strengthen a weak group of muscles by repetition of movements, the patient is shown how to stretch the tightened muscles, thereby encouraging the weak ones to strengthen.

### Natural medicines

Certain natural medicines can help to stimulate physiological changes in the body, thus relieving pain. Natural plant-based remedies prescribed by homeopaths (see page 85) and herbalists (see page 86) are particularly suitable for pain caused by internal disorders affecting the lungs, digestive system and urinary tract.

Other natural medicines can be used as physical stimuli to relieve pain. For example, naturopaths often prescribe hot or cold compresses to provide counter-irritation. This works by overloading the pain gate and causing it to close, thus preventing the further transmission of pain messages (see page 18). Naturopaths also advise on nutritional and dietary strategies to reduce susceptibility to pain.

### MIND TRAINING

Research has shown that the mind can help to stimulate the body's natural defence mechanisms to assist in healing and relieving pain. An understanding of the part played by the mind in the overall experience of pain can enable you to actively decrease the amount of pain you suffer. If you are discontented or unhappy you are more likely to be unhealthy and less able to deal effectively with pain; conversely mental well-being and joy have a positive effect on the body's ability to cope with pain. Visualisation is one technique that uses this principle. By imagining being in a peaceful country setting, for example, you can help yourself to relax and reduce the stress that might otherwise hinder the healing process.

Other therapies aim to calm the emotions by resolving conflicts which may be at the root of some pains. Headaches, for example, can often be the product of tensions created by unresolved or deep-rooted anxieties. Various forms of psychotherapy (see page 89) can help the patient to resolve these or come to terms with them, and ultimately pain relief can be achieved.

### Relaxation therapies

Wherever pain is located in the body and whatever its nature, either physical or emotional, the ability to relax and have good quality sleep are essential to its relief. Damaged or inflamed tissues are also repaired more efficiently during sleep as the blood releases greater levels of hormones which promote regeneration and healing.

Even sitting quietly, perhaps listening to soothing music, can be beneficial as it rests the body and distracts the mind, but for many people the more focused approach of relaxation techniques (see page 91) is more effective at releasing tension in the skeletal muscles. Relaxing the muscles eases the over-stimulation of the nerves and alleviates the mental tension that this can cause.

The ability to let go physically is quite natural during early childhood but as we grow up we develop bad postural habits and suffer injuries and emotional trauma. All of these contribute to muscle tension, circulation problems and – according to Eastern philosophy – the blockage of energy flows which lead to pain. Many of the techniques described in the following pages suggest ways of reducing these tensions and so unblocking obstructions to good health.

**Pain clinics**

If conventional treatments have been tried without success, your doctor may refer you to a pain clinic. Pain clinics may employ a mix of complementary and orthodox approaches to pain management. These may include pain-killing injections such as epidurals (see page 120), behavioural psychology, autogenic training (see page 88) or biofeedback (see page 92). Some clinics offer a range of complementary treatments, such as acupuncture, Alexander Technique, osteopathy, chiropractic and aromatherapy.

# Manipulative Therapies

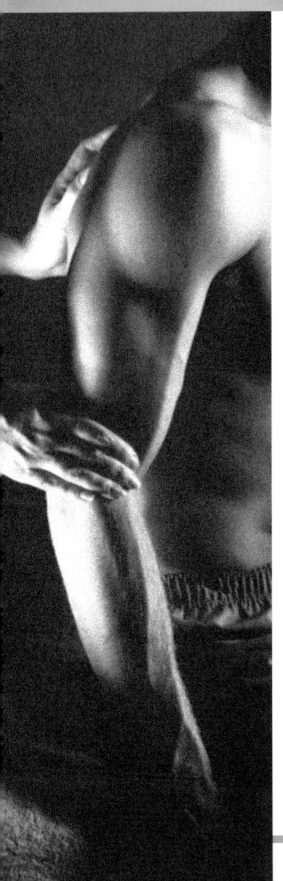

*Manipulative treatments work with the muscles and skeleton to alleviate backache and other muscle and joint pain. By restoring balance to the body, these treatments can provide long-term relief from pain due to such causes as bad posture or arthritis.*

## CHIROPRACTIC

Chiropractic is based on the theory that pain is caused by some dysfunction of the musculoskeletal system. The treatment involves manipulation of the body joints in order to restore normal nerve function, alleviate pain and improve muscle efficiency. Chiropractors focus their manual skills principally on the spinal column. If the range of movement of spinal joints is even slightly displaced or restricted, it can cause considerable pain in the back, arms, or legs. Displaced vertebrae press on the tissues surrounding the nerves that pass out of the spinal cord and can cause pain locally or along the pathway of the affected nerve, as in sciatica. There can also be pain or muscle spasm round the affected joint. Misaligned vertebrae are called 'subluxations'.

**Method** A chiropractor will try to mobilise and release the restrictions of the spinal joints. The treatment may involve sharp, rapid thrusts and other mobilising techniques that act directly on the affected joints. This kind of treatment is particularly beneficial for problems connected with the spine such as sciatica and backache. Chiropractic may also be beneficial in other disorders. If you suffer from migraines, for example, a chiropractor may make adjustments to the atlas and axis bones at the top of the spinal column to help to

alleviate the pain. For chest or abdomen problems, you may find that the chiropractor pays particular attention to the thoracic vertebrae (between the neck and the waist). This is because the joints of this area enable free movement of the ribs and respiratory muscles. In addition, important nerves to and from the abdominal organs pass between the vertebrae in this area. A variety of techniques may be used on the skin, muscles and connective tissue.

**Result** Some patients experience immediate relief from pain but more often the pain is relieved gradually as the joints become more flexible. Others suffer slight stiffness and soreness at first before the treatment is effective. Several treatments may be necessary before pain is alleviated.

### HOW IT CAN HELP

*Chiropractic treatment makes small adjustments to the spine which in turn can improve the function of the joints, muscles, ligaments and nerves all over the body. The treatment is useful for:*

▶ Arthritic pain and stiffness

▶ Neck and back pain

▶ Shoulder, knee and other joint injuries

▶ Sciatica and neuralgia

▶ Headaches and migraine

# OSTEOPATHY

Osteopathy was first developed by Andrew Taylor Still and arose partly from his experiences as a surgeon treating injured soldiers during the American Civil War. Similar in aim to chiropractic, osteopathy aims to ease displaced or restricted joints and muscles which may be causing pain or interfering with normal function. Osteopathy is effective at relieving pain caused by a variety of conditions such as arthritis, rheumatism and migraine.

**Method** Osteopathic treatment uses manual procedures to stretch and loosen the muscles and ligaments, with gentle manipulation of the joints to restore their normal range of movement. Practitioners may use a manipulation movement known as the 'thrust technique' which aims to improve the mobility of a joint.

Although osteopathy and chiropractic have much in common, osteopathic manipulation tends to be less direct than chiropractic adjustments. Rather than manipulating the spine directly, osteopaths focus on the limbs and trunk to improve the movement of the joint. Osteopaths also work on other joints such as the knees, ankles, elbows, shoulders and wrists.

An important element of osteopathic treatment is the manipulation of the soft tissues – the muscles, ligaments and connective tissues which surround and support the joints. The neuromuscular technique, a special type of soft-tissue therapy used by some osteopaths, is effective in relieving pain associated with abnormal thickening of muscles and ligaments. Muscle tension in the neck, shoulders and upper back can cause a great deal of pain but can be alleviated by neuromuscular techniques combined with osteopathic manipulation.

**Result** After osteopathic treatment the relief from some back and neck problems is noticeable straightaway, especially if a restricted joint is successfully freed. More commonly, however, there is a gradual reduction of pain with regular treatment over successive weeks or months. Research has shown that it is particularly beneficial for the treatment of lower back pain.

## HOW IT CAN HELP

*Osteopathic treatment is particularly effective for:*

► Arthritic stiffness and pain
► Neck and back pain
► Headaches and migraine
► Neuralgia of the face and jaw
► Shoulder, arm and leg pains, for example 'frozen shoulder', sciatica, 'tennis elbow'
► Sports injuries

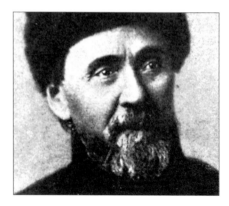

*ANDREW TAYLOR STILL (1828–1917) The founder of osteopathy, A.T. Still said his technique could also treat infections and degenerative disorders – a claim not made by osteopaths today.*

## CRANIAL OSTEOPATHY

At the beginning of the century osteopaths discovered that the bones and binding tissues of the skull and spinal column are not entirely static. Even when the body is resting there is a constant rhythmical motion in the cranial bones which coordinates with a subtle undulation of the spinal column and sacral bone. Disturbances of these rhythmical movements may lead to headaches, migraines, and other neuralgic conditions of the face and jaw. These stiff parts of the skull can be gently manipulated by an osteopath to regain their flexibility. Cranial techniques are increasingly being used with babies and children suffering from birth or developmental problems, for example, resulting from a difficult forceps delivery.

*RESTORING CRANIAL RHYTHMS The cranial osteopath cradles the patient's skull and with gentle movements restores healthier patterns of motion to stiff and restricted areas.*

# ROLFING

Rolfing is a type of deep-tissue manipulation developed in the 1940s by Dr Ida Rolf, a US doctor. She questioned the belief that postural well-being was solely dependent on the bones and directed her treatment at the muscles and connective tissues. She found that connective tissue often became distorted to compensate for bad posture habits. By stretching and manipulating the connective tissues, she believed that she could restore the body's balance and alignment.

**Method** In common with other structural practitioners, a rolfer will first check for any distortions in your posture. The practitioner will then start treatment using the knuckles and fingers to stretch and separate layers of muscles and connective tissues. The work usually begins around the neck, shoulders and rib cage, moving on to the feet, legs, pelvis and back in a systematic way.

**Result** Rolfing is a vigorous and deep form of soft-tissue massage which some patients may find rather uncomfortable initially. However, it can be highly effective in releasing chronically stiffened muscles. Many people feel a great emotional release after rolfing treatment.

## HOW IT CAN HELP

*Rolfing is particularly useful for patients suffering from pain brought about by poor posture. Its ability to maintain the body's natural alignment makes it a valuable preventative treatment. It is also useful for:*

▶ Headaches, especially those due to tension and stiffness of the neck and shoulders

▶ Chronic pain in the back, neck, and limbs due to occupational stresses, both physical and mental

▶ Chronic joint pains and disorders resulting from poor posture

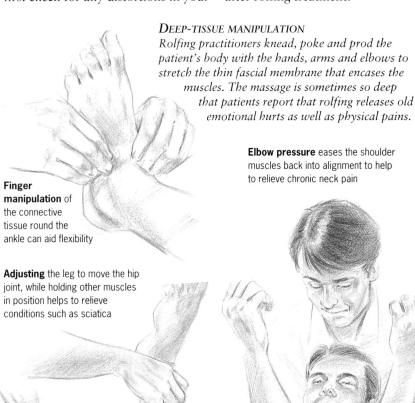

*DEEP-TISSUE MANIPULATION*
*Rolfing practitioners knead, poke and prod the patient's body with the hands, arms and elbows to stretch the thin fascial membrane that encases the muscles. The massage is sometimes so deep that patients report that rolfing releases old emotional hurts as well as physical pains.*

**Finger manipulation** of the connective tissue round the ankle can aid flexibility

**Adjusting** the leg to move the hip joint, while holding other muscles in position helps to relieve conditions such as sciatica

**Elbow pressure** eases the shoulder muscles back into alignment to help to relieve chronic neck pain

## Origins

Rolfing was named after its founder Dr Ida Rolf an American biochemist and physiologist. She first became interested in body structure when she was treated by an osteopath after being kicked by a horse. The system she devised, which she called 'structural integration', combined her knowledge of yoga with manipulation techniques.

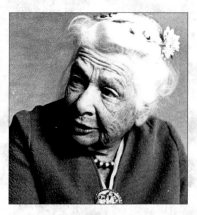

*IDA ROLF (1896–1976)*
*Dr Ida Rolf developed her techniques as a way to bring the body back into physical alignment with the Earth's gravitational pull.*

## PHYSIOTHERAPY

Physiotherapists use a wide range of techniques for dealing with pain and muscle and joint problems. Massage features strongly, and treatments such as heat therapy, ultrasound, electrotherapy and exercise are also widely used.

**Method** Disorders of the musculo-skeletal system may be treated with massage and careful manipulation of the joints, often in conjunction with a structured programme of exercises. Practitioners may use heat packs or infra-red lamps to relieve painful muscle spasms or assist healing, and cold treatment, such as the application of ice packs, to reduce inflammation and swelling.

Physiotherapists are skilled in the use of a range of sophisticated electrical techniques. These include ultrasound to reduce inflammation, and transcutaneous electrical nerve stimulation (TENS) to relieve pain. A form of deep heat treatment called diathermy, using high-frequency electrical currents, can reduce the pain of conditions such as

rheumatism or arthritis. Such treatments can also promote healing by improving the blood supply to, and lymphatic drainage from, the muscles and connective tissues.

**Result** Physiotherapy techniques can prevent or reduce joint stiffness and alleviate the pain caused by inflammation and muscle spasm. Physiotherapy can reduce pain and accelerate healing and is particularly effective at restoring limb function, joint mobility and muscle strength after injury, major surgery or stroke.

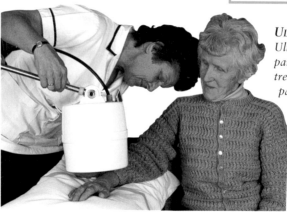

*ULTRASOUND*
*Ultrasound has proved particularly effective in the treatment of soft-tissue injuries, particularly involving ligaments, muscles and tendons round the joints. It works by improving blood flow to the damaged tissues and so accelerating the healing process and reducing inflammation.*

## METAMORPHIC TECHNIQUE

Metamorphic technique is a gentle and relaxing form of treatment involving fingertip pressure on the feet. It was originally devised to treat disturbed and handicapped children, but is now used for people of all ages and conditions. It is based on the belief that the foot corresponds to the development of the foetus between conception and birth. Practitioners believe that all human patterns of behaviour and responses, whether physical, mental, emotional or spiritual, are set in the womb, mainly arising from the mother's mental condition at the time. Metamorphic technique links the foot with the organs and other structures of the body, especially

with the spine and the head. The practitioner aims to act as a catalyst, enabling patients to use their innate healing ability to help themselves.

**Method** The practitioner lightly touches various reflex points on the foot running along a line starting at the big toe and extending over the arch of the foot to the heel. By pressing points close to the toes, the practitioner treats traumas arising during the early development of the foetus. Traumas arising during later development in the womb are treated by pressing points farther along the foot or on the heel itself. The practitioner may also touch points on the hands and the back of the head.

**Result** Patients report feeling relaxed with more vitality and an enhanced sense of well-being. However, as the aim of metamorphic technique is to enable patients to heal themselves, the lasting effects may be seen only over the longer term.

# Movement Therapies

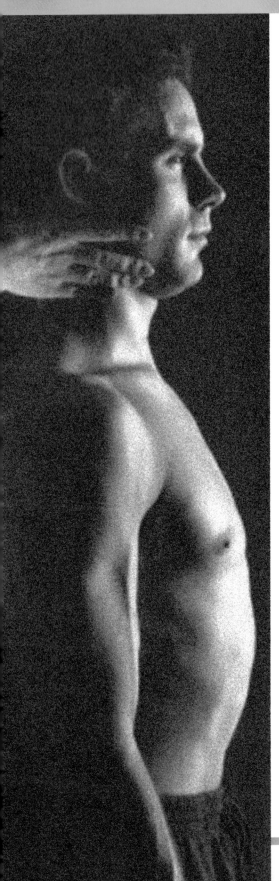

*Awareness of your body's posture – the way you stand, sit, and move in everyday activities – is important for the prevention of muscle and joint pain and some stress disorders. Posture and exercise can improve coordination and aid relaxation.*

## YOGA

Yoga, from the Sanskrit word for 'union', originated in India more than 4000 years ago. There are many forms of yoga being practised today, ranging from the mainly physical systems of exercise to those which also emphasise the original meditative and spiritual aspects.

**Method** Hatha yoga, the type most commonly taught in the West, is a blend of postures, breathing, and meditation. The yoga postures, or asanas, aim to keep the body supple and consist mainly of stretching and bending movements performed very slowly in time with the breathing. During a yoga session asanas are performed in standing, sitting and lying positions, followed by a period of relaxation. Yoga can be practised by people of all ages and fitness levels, although you will be advised to avoid positions which are difficult to achieve or cause discomfort.

**Result** People who practise yoga regularly develop greater physical flexibility and mental serenity, which can help them to cope with chronic painful conditions.

*YOGA TO EASE TENSION*
*Yoga exercises are particularly useful for relieving pain and other symptoms associated with stress and depression.*

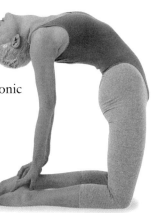

### HOW IT CAN HELP

*Yoga has been found to be beneficial for both chronic pain and as part of a therapeutic programme for patients suffering from stress-related disorders. It is particularly recommended for patients with:*

▶ High blood pressure

▶ Headaches, migraines

▶ Severe chronic pain such as arthritis

▶ Asthma

▶ Bronchitis

▶ Painful periods

▶ Depression

▶ Stomach disorders

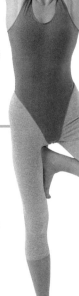

# T'AI CHI AND QIGONG

T'ai chi (pronounced 'tie-chee') is a system of coordinated exercises which originated in China as a refined version of martial arts such as kung fu. The name means 'the supreme unity' and the aim is to develop coordination and muscular control rather than muscle strength.

Qigong (pronounced 'chee-gong'), is a more vigorous type of movement with similar aims. The name means 'manipulation of vital energy'. Both forms of therapy are concerned not simply with physical exercise but with achieving well-being by harmonising the flow of energy (known as chi or qi) along special pathways within the body.

**Method** T'ai chi consists of a series of circular, flowing movements that are coordinated with carefully managed breathing patterns and performed quite slowly. Qigong uses a system of breathing exercises combined with postures and movements to achieve deep concentration.

Unlike yoga, where many postures are practised while sitting on the floor, t'ai chi and qigong are performed in a standing position. The feet move slowly in a sequence of steps while the arms and upper body rotate gently through a range of movements symbolically 'gathering' and 'channelling' energy. Teachers of qigong may also use their hands and fingers to transmit energy to acupuncture points.

T'ai chi and qigong have a spiritual dimension, sometimes being described as 'moving meditation'. The sequence of movements take some time to learn so it is best to join a class until you develop confidence.

## HOW IT CAN HELP

*In addition to improving general well-being the following conditions can be helped in the longer term with regular practice:*
- ▶ Headaches
- ▶ Neck and shoulder aches
- ▶ Lower back pain
- ▶ Angina

**Result** T'ai chi and qigong are both excellent exercise therapies for boosting energy levels and reducing stress. Exercise sessions can easily be fitted into any spare time you have during the day. They are particularly well suited to people with physical disorders resulting from a stressful working life, such as headaches, migraines, and neck, shoulder and back pain.

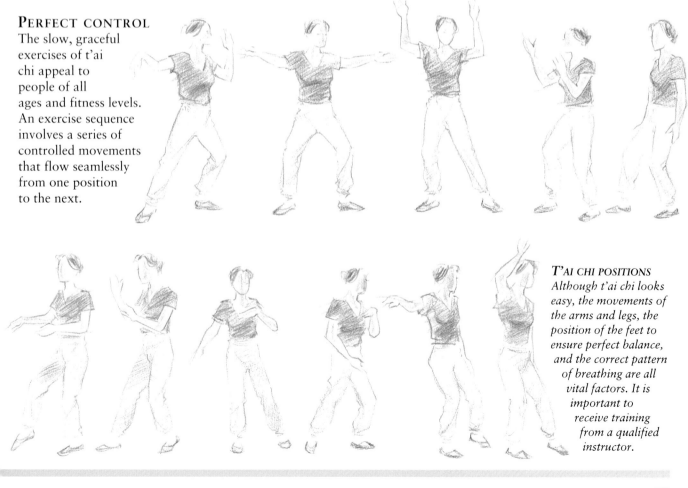

**PERFECT CONTROL**
The slow, graceful exercises of t'ai chi appeal to people of all ages and fitness levels. An exercise sequence involves a series of controlled movements that flow seamlessly from one position to the next.

*T'AI CHI POSITIONS*
*Although t'ai chi looks easy, the movements of the arms and legs, the position of the feet to ensure perfect balance, and the correct pattern of breathing are all vital factors. It is important to receive training from a qualified instructor.*

# ALEXANDER TECHNIQUE

The Alexander Technique is a system of postural re-education developed by Frederick Alexander. He believed that many disorders of the muscles and skeleton were the result of stresses caused by poor posture habits. Manipulation and massage were not sufficient to correct misalignment, he believed. It was necessary to learn how to use the body correctly, not just to relieve painful symptoms but to prevent such problems recurring.

**Method** Alexander Technique can only be learned effectively from a qualified teacher who will help you to become aware of poor postural habits. The teacher will encourage you to develop what Alexander himself called 'conscious self-awareness' to identify what is wrong with your sitting, standing and walking posture. Unsuitable patterns will then be corrected gradually. Your Alexander teacher will also show you postural exercises which you can do at home.

**Result** New ways of sitting or moving can feel strange when you are used to the old faulty ones, so be aware that it takes time to correct defects in posture. Once any pain is alleviated, Alexander teachers recommend you perform simple exercises to maintain the beneficial effect.

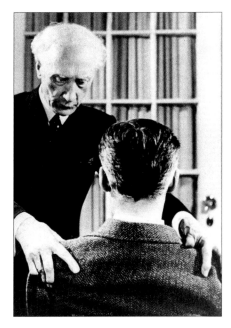

## HOW IT CAN HELP

*Alexander Technique is first and foremost a preventative approach, but it is also effective in relieving pain caused by musculoskeletal problems and related disorders. It is particularly useful for:*

▶ Neck and shoulder problems, particularly among musicians such as violinists and pianists

▶ Recurrent sports-related disorders, such as tennis elbow

▶ Recurrent back pain and sciatica

▶ Chronic conditions such as asthma and headaches

▶ Facial neuralgia

▶ Osteoarthritis

## IMPROVING POSTURE
The way you sit and stand can contribute to back and neck pain, as well as other conditions. By ensuring correct posture you can help to avoid musculoskeletal disorders.

*THE ALEXANDER TOUCH*
*F.M. Alexander was an Australian actor who became interested in the role of posture in health. He developed a system of exercises to treat a range of disorders. Although the technique may be difficult to learn initially it can be very beneficial for reducing muscular and mental tension. Many people find the technique helpful for rehabilitation after back and neck injuries. Once you have learnt the technique from a professional you can practise the exercises at home.*

*GETTING UP*
**1** *When getting out of a chair, always aim to bend at the hips, knees and ankles only. Try to keep your neck and spine in alignment at all times. Try not to push your head too far forward when you rise as this gives the spine an unhealthy curvature.*

*STANDING UP*
**2** *As you stand and straighten, bring your head, spine and legs into alignment, as though being lifted by a wire attached to the top of your head. Avoid slouching forward or holding your shoulders too far back – both can lead to back and neck aches and pains.*

# FELDENKRAIS

Feldenkrais is a system of movement and postural retraining developed by Dr Moshe Feldenkrais, a Russian-born physicist. He developed two related techniques: 'awareness through movement', often taught in classes, and individual tuition using gentle manipulation which he termed 'functional integration'.

**Method** A Feldenkrais practitioner will encourage you to become more aware of your posture by gradually stimulating the nerve and muscle coordination with new patterns of movement. You will then be led through a series of gentle movements designed to help the breakdown of muscular patterns established through years of misuse. If you are suffering from severe pain, Feldenkrais teachers recommend the one-to-one approach of functional integration. In this technique the practitioner will move your joints manually through a range of movements. Instead of working directly on the painful joint, such as the shoulder, however, your teacher may tackle the problem through another limb, perhaps the leg. This transmits impulses to the brain, helping it to learn new patterns of movement so that the damaged area of the body can be moved more efficiently.

**Result** Once the main problems have been dealt with, Feldenkrais instructors recommend simple exercise (see page 59). Additional benefits noted by patients include improved breathing, circulation and general health.

## HOW IT CAN HELP

*The gentle movements in Feldenkrais therapy are useful for patients suffering from recurring muscle and joint pain. It has been found particularly beneficial for improving brain and muscle coordination and so is popular among those whose lives involve a lot of movement, such as athletes, musicians, dancers. The technique is also an efficient preventative therapy, helping to reduce the risk of injury by teaching efficient muscle use. It is most useful for:*

- ► Arthritis and osteoarthritis
- ► Chronic backache and spinal disorders
- ► Rehabilitation after a stroke
- ► Cerebral palsy
- ► Children with learning problems

# PILATES

The Pilates method is a system of rehabilitation through non-weight-bearing or non-impact exercise. In contrast to osteopathy and chiropractic which emphasise 'stretching the strong to strengthen the weak', Pilates exercises isolate and strengthen weaker muscles but without overdeveloping strong ones.

**Method** The programme will be tailored to your ability and needs. You will be placed carefully in the lying position on a specially designed couch and then asked to perform a series of exercises. The movements are designed to isolate muscular imbalances, strengthen weak muscles, and relax over-developed muscles. The exercises also help to mobilise the joints and release tension. The movements are slow and controlled, emphasising natural evolution rather than a forced change. Your instructor will show you specific breathing techniques for each exercise that help direct energy to the working areas while relaxing the rest of the body.

**Result** By correcting imbalances, much of the pain associated with disorders of the musculoskeletal system is avoided. After treatment, patients report improved muscle control, flexibility, coordination, strength and tone. The system is particularly helpful when combined with treatment by other manipulative therapists.

## HOW IT CAN HELP

*Regular supervised sessions of the Pilates method can prevent much of the pain caused by lower back ailments. It is beneficial for:*

- ► Rehabilitation after surgery
- ► Regaining fitness after illness
- ► Maintaining general good health
- ► Arthritis
- ► Lower back pain and tension in the upper back
- ► Rheumatism
- ► Osteoporosis
- ► Injuries to the muscles and joints, particularly involving the knee, ankle, foot and shoulder

*BACK THERAPY*
*Pilates exercises can tackle problems such as lower back pain by strengthening muscles in the legs, arms and other parts of the body.*

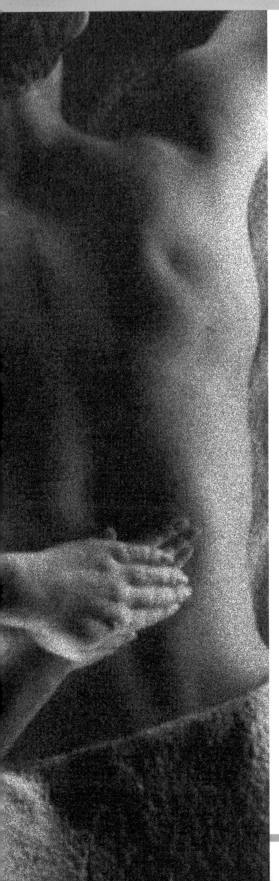

# Massage Therapies

*Massage offers a relaxing and pleasurable way of dealing with pain and is widely available in a variety of forms, some based on Oriental medicine. The basic techniques of massage are easy to learn and can be used to give pain relief to family and friends.*

## MASSAGE

Massage (from the French word 'masser', meaning 'to rub') is one of the oldest therapies known. It may have developed from the discovery that simply rubbing a sore area provides immediate relief. As it became evident that rubbing relieved not only local pains but also those in other parts of the body, the value of using the hands for healing must have been realised and more systematic approaches developed.

**Method** Basic massage consists of stroking, kneading, tapping and stretching movements made mainly in the direction of the heart. By manipulating the soft tissues of the body, massage can relieve muscle tension and so provide mental and physical relaxation. Stimulating the skin with massage techniques is also believed to improve blood flow towards the centre of the body and thus improve circulation.

Massage is useful for alleviating pain caused by sports injuries and is also frequently used in rehabilitation programmes for patients who have had an accident or stroke. A practitioner pays particular attention to the muscles and tendons in the area of an injury, such as the back or leg, to relieve stiffness and pain.

Massage is also a convenient way of applying therapeutic substances to the skin and underlying tissues. Many sports masseurs use warming

### HOW IT CAN HELP

*Massage can help to relieve muscular pain as well as reducing stress and easing muscle tension. The treatment is useful for:*

▶ Relieving neck and back pain

▶ Aiding relaxation

▶ Mobilising stiff joints

▶ Improving muscle tone

▶ Stimulating release of endorphins, the body's natural painkillers

▶ Helping the healing process by improving the supply of oxygen and nutrients to the muscles and connective tissues

▶ Improving drainage of waste products from the tissues

or analgesic creams and oils, while aromatherapy massage uses a variety of essential oils.

**Result** Many people have regular massage to help them to relax and stay in peak physical condition. Those engaged in physically active pursuits, such as dancers and footballers, find it particularly useful for maintaining muscle tone. Massage also has valuable preventative health benefits as it improves the flexibility of muscles and connective tissue and enhances their blood supply, and also helps to boost the body's immune system.

## MASSAGE STROKES

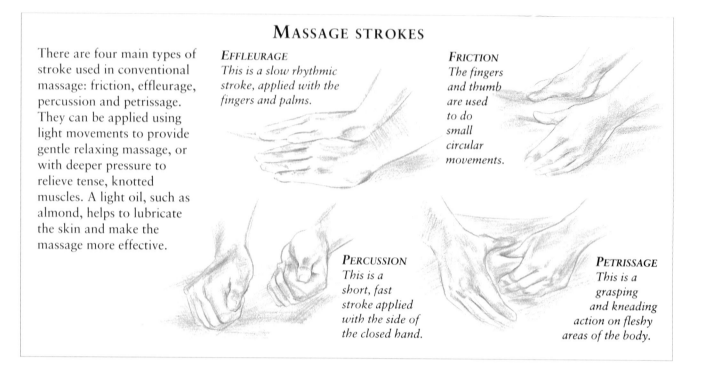

There are four main types of stroke used in conventional massage: friction, effleurage, percussion and petrissage. They can be applied using light movements to provide gentle relaxing massage, or with deeper pressure to relieve tense, knotted muscles. A light oil, such as almond, helps to lubricate the skin and make the massage more effective.

*EFFLEURAGE*
*This is a slow rhythmic stroke, applied with the fingers and palms.*

*FRICTION*
*The fingers and thumb are used to do small circular movements.*

*PERCUSSION*
*This is a short, fast stroke applied with the side of the closed hand.*

*PETRISSAGE*
*This is a grasping and kneading action on fleshy areas of the body.*

## AROMATHERAPY

In aromatherapy, oils with healing properties, known as 'essential oils', are used as a compress or steam inhalation, added to bath water, or massaged into the skin. Essential oils are extracted from various medicinal plants by a process of distillation. They are highly concentrated so only a few drops are needed. For a massage, a few drops of one or more essential oils are added to a carrier or base oil, such as almond oil.

Essential oils are absorbed into the body by inhalation and through the skin. They can have a localised effect and also pass into the bloodstream to reach other areas of the body. Some oils affect mood, for example, by relieving tension or depression. Aromatherapy is useful for treating stress-related disorders, and chronic painful conditions such as arthritis.

**Method** Essential oils are available from chemists or health stores for use at home, but for treatment that is tailored to your personal condition, it is advisable to visit a trained aromatherapist. After a discussion of your condition, the aromatherapist will select oils that you can use at home or will offer to apply them by massage. For the relief of respiratory disorders such as bronchitis, or sinusitis, the therapist will provide a combination of oils to be added to hot water for a steam inhalation.

**Result** As well as alleviating some specific disorders, aromatherapy aids relaxation and promotes the release of endorphins, thereby providing relief from conditions such as anxiety, and muscle and joint pain.

### HOW IT CAN HELP

*Aromatherapy can ease stress-related disorders and emotional states such as anxiety and depression. It is also helpful in alleviating:*

▶ Nasal congestion and sinusitis (in a steam inhalation)
▶ Muscular tension
▶ Chronic neck and back pain
▶ High blood pressure
▶ Premenstrual symptoms
▶ Chronic bronchitis

### MASSAGE OILS

You can buy massage oils ready mixed, or you can make your own by buying essential oils and mixing a few drops with a base oil, such as almond or hazelnut oil. Essential oils should be kept in cool, dark surroundings, but not in the fridge as cold can degrade the quality of the oil.

*ESSENTIAL OILS*
*Keep essential oils in glass bottles with tight-fitting stoppers.*

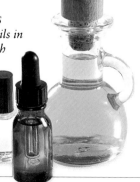

# Energy Therapies

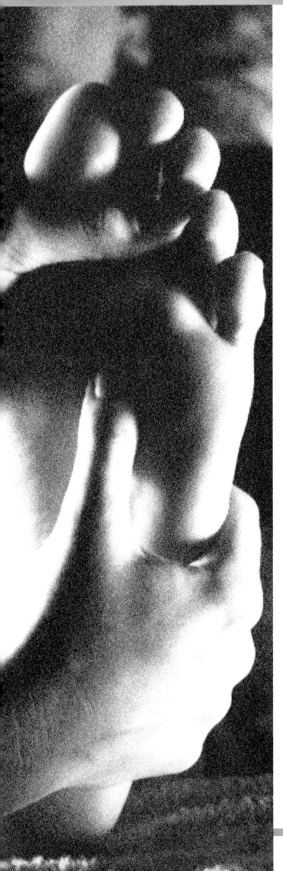

*Many treatments are based on the theory that energy pathways in the body play a part in health and well-being. Any blockages, deficiencies or imbalances in these pathways cause symptoms. Treatment aims to restore the energy flow to a state of harmony.*

## ACUPUNCTURE

Acupuncture and several other Oriental disciplines, such as shiatsu and acupressure, are based on the traditional Chinese theory that pain and illness are the result of an excess or deficiency of energy, 'chi' or 'qi', in the affected area of the body. The body's energy flows through a network of channels, or 'meridians', that are said to lie just below the body's surface. These meridians connect specific organs and systems, and have a wider sphere of influence in the body. Acupuncturists focus on special points on the meridians to correct imbalances in the energy flow and thus relieve pain and illness.

In China acupuncture is often used as an anaesthetic during surgical operations, providing complete pain relief while the patient remains awake. It is becoming a widely popular method of pain relief during labour as it has no effect on the baby and allows the mother to remain alert throughout the birth.

**Method**  The principal tools of acupuncture are fine stainless steel or silver alloy needles. These are inserted into the skin at the specific acupuncture points. This is a painless procedure, the only sensation being a slight tingling as the needle reaches the chosen point. The needles may be inserted in a variety of ways from vertically to almost horizontally. The acupuncturist may rotate or manipulate the needles to give added stimulation to the point. Sometimes a mild electric current is sent through a needle to achieve the same effect.

The acupuncturist may burn a small cone of a dried herb, usually mugwort (*Artemisia vulgaris*) or moxa (*Artemisia japonica*), over the point, or hold the glowing end of a moxa stick close to the point. Or a piece of moxa may be placed on the head of the needle and set alight. The smouldering moxa imparts a gentle heat down the shaft of the needle into the energy channel.

**Result**  Pain relief through acupuncture can be almost instantaneous; other patients report improvements after several sessions. Acupuncture has often proved particularly effective for the relief of pain caused by arthritic joints and stiff muscles.

---

### HOW IT CAN HELP

*Acupuncture is effective at easing chronic pain and also for alleviating stress-related conditions. It is particularly suited to the treatment of:*

► Arthritis
► Rheumatism
► Angina
► Digestive disorders
► Fatigue

## ACUPRESSURE

In this therapy gentle pressure is applied to the acupuncture points with the fingertips or a blunt probe. Acupressure follows similar principles to those of acupuncture but may, in fact, predate it. It is likely that acupuncture points were first discovered by massaging and pressing tender areas on the body. The earliest medical tools discovered at archaeological sites in China are blunt-pointed pebbles, known as the 'bian stones', which might have been used before the advent of needles. Acupressure is safe to use as a self-help treatment for many common ailments, such as travel sickness.

**Method** Acupressure has the same aim as acupuncture, to restore the flow of energy along the meridians and to release any blockages. Treatment consists of sustaining firm pressure on selected acupuncture points for up to a minute or more, or stimulating the points using a circular, kneading movement. Pressure is usually applied with the fingertips or thumbs but can also be done with a rounded probe such as a pen top.

**Result** Many people have reported relief from a range of symptoms including arthritis, back pain, and

digestive and circulation problems. It has also proved effective in the self-treatment of conditions such as migraine and tension.

### HOW IT CAN HELP

*Acupressure is an excellent preventative treatment. It is also useful for specific painful ailments such as:*

▶ Headaches and migraine
▶ Backache
▶ Digestive problems
▶ Chronic stiffness
▶ Sports injuries

## REIKI

Reiki aims to re-balance the energy in the body to stimulate the body's natural healing systems and achieve greater well-being. It was developed in 19th-century Japan by a spiritual master, Dr Mikao Usui, to harmonise body energy with the energy of its surroundings. The term 'reiki' is the Japanese for 'universal energy'.

**Method** Reiki is really a form of meditation based on the concept that the body radiates a vital life force or energy. Reiki healers must first 'attune' themselves to this life energy to give them the ability to heal others. Once attuned the healer then learns a range of hand positions to use for self treatment, the treatment of others and for group healing.

At a healing session you will be asked to lie on a massage table. The therapist will then place his or her hands on or above the body at points believed to be emitting weak energy. The hands are held palms down with the fingers and thumbs extended and held together. The treatment is gentle but powerful, stimulating the body's self-healing ability.

**Result** After receiving reiki therapy, the patient usually feels a relaxing warmth and sometimes even a pleasant tingling sensation. It can also help people bring deep-seated emotional problems to the fore so that they can be resolved.

*GROUP HEALING*
*Traditional Japanese Reiki healers worked in teams, which makes the healing session much faster as several hand positions can be performed at once. A team can consist of as many as eight or nine healers.*

### HOW IT CAN HELP

*Reiki is said to be of benefit in a wide range of disorders. It is effective at calming the nervous system and so is often used in combination with other techniques as part of a pain management programme. It is particularly useful for easing the pain associated with:*

▶ Stress-related disorders
▶ Chronic neck and back pain
▶ Period pain
▶ Chronic joint disorders

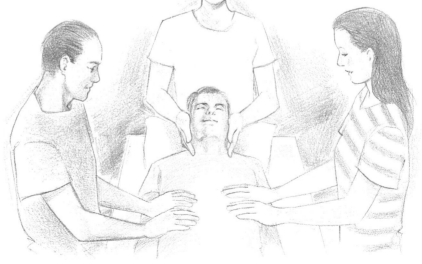

## KINESIOLOGY

Kinesiology was developed by Dr George Goodheart, an American chiropractor. Its original aim was to treat muscular imbalances which can result in poor posture and pain. It is widely used by chiropractors and osteopaths, some of whom have evolved their own variations to diagnose and treat many health problems. Some practitioners practise kinesiology exclusively while others use it as an adjunct to osteopathy or chiropractic work.

The principle behind the standard form of kinesiology is that weakness of specific muscles, with the consequent changes in posture, are responsible for causing pain. Practitioners believe that the weak muscles create an imbalance in the body's energy channels, or meridians. Some 'indicator' muscles are said to be linked to these meridians and can provide information about the whole body.

**Method** A kinesiologist will first check your posture and then examine you in standing and sitting positions, looking for muscular imbalances. There may, for example, be a tilt of the head or a dropped shoulder on one side. The practitioner will then carry out tests on individual muscles while you are in a standing, sitting or lying position by applying light pressure to their normal action for a few seconds and gauging their relative strength.

The way the muscles respond to the tests reveals to the practitioner how the body is functioning. For example, strong resistance is a sign of health and poor resistance is a sign of weakness. These tests rely on the practitioner's knowledge of the muscles' actions and relationships. Strong muscles that weaken after an unsuitable food is placed in the mouth can be used as indicators of food intolerance.

### HOW IT CAN HELP

*Kinesiology is best suited for locating and correcting physical disorders and thus is most effective in treating or preventing:*

▶ Muscular and joint pains due to distorted posture

▶ Joint inflammation

▶ Headache, migraine and neuralgia

If a problem area is identified, the kinesiologist will gently massage the acupoints, or trigger points, in the muscles with the fingertips to try to revitalise the area.

**Result** Kinesiology provides a picture of your general state of health. Many patients report increased vitality and energy after treatment. The treatment is also well suited as a preventative measure.

## SHIATSU

Shiatsu is a Japanese therapy, with roots in Chinese medicine, which is based on the belief that stimulating points on the surface of the body can influence the functioning of organs deep inside. As in acupressure, shiatsu works by the application of pressure to acupuncture points in order to stimulate the body's energy flow and remove any blockages from the energy channels or meridians. It also incorporates massage techniques to treat a wide range of disorders. The pressure points are located along the meridians at places where the energy channels lie close to the skin.

**Method** The name shiatsu comes from the Japanese for 'finger massage'. The practitioner uses circular motions and firm pressure applied with the fingertips and thumbs to specific energy points or along the course of the energy channels. Sometimes practitioners use the heels of their hands, their elbows, knees and even their feet to apply suitable pressure. The strength of the pressure depends on the location and on whether the aim is to stimulate or sedate the energy flow. Light stroking techniques are used where energy is congested, and sustained or stronger pressure is applied to stimulate the skin.

Where there is pain in a specific area such as the knee, the energy flow may be sluggish so the aim of treatment is to clear the obstruction. For a painful joint, the practitioner will focus not only on the joint itself but also on points along the energy channels that pass through the affected area, which may lie some distance away from the actual location of the pain.

### HOW IT CAN HELP

*Like acupressure, shiatsu is an effective preventative treatment and is useful for specific painful ailments such as:*

▶ Headaches and migraine

▶ Musculoskeletal disorders

▶ Digestive problems

▶ Bowel disorders

▶ Sports injuries

**Result** Shiatsu has proved most effective for the relief of tension and other stress-related conditions, and musculoskeletal disorders such as chronic neck and back pain. Patients often report an increased vitality and release from depression and insomnia. Shiatsu is also believed to prevent disease by strengthening the body's immune system.

# REFLEXOLOGY

Reflexology involves fingertip pressure on areas on the feet called 'reflex zones' in order to relieve pain in other parts of the body. The technique is thought to have originated in China over 5000 years ago. Reflexology was revived and developed by a New York therapist, Eunice Ingham, in the 1930s. She discovered that certain areas, mainly on the soles of the feet, but also on the hands, appeared to correspond to organs and regions of the body. Tenderness of individual foot zones coincided with disturbance of the corresponding organ. Pain in an area of the body such as the head or the abdomen can be relieved by working on the corresponding foot zone. Reflexology is now widely practised in conjunction with other therapies and many people have learnt it in order to help family and friends.

**Method** The reflexologist uses the thumb and fingers to stimulate the reflex points. If the person receiving the treatment has a serious health problem, applying any pressure can sometimes be quite painful. Sessions of reflexology treatment generally last about an hour.

**Result** Patients often report that a session with a reflexologist can provide a huge energy boost, as well as relaxing the body and bringing it back into balance. It is sometimes possible to practise the technique at home, but patients should take the advice of a practitioner before treating themselves.

## HOW IT CAN HELP

*Reflexology is better suited for general disorders and stress-related problems rather than specific conditions. It is useful for:*

► Migraines, tension and fatigue
► Digestive problems, such as constipation
► Period pains

# TENS (TRANSCUTANEOUS ELECTRICAL NERVE STIMULATION)

The idea of using electrotherapy to alleviate pain dates back to Roman times when a live electric eel was used to ease the pain of gout. TENS is a modern version of electrotherapy that spans both physical and energy approaches. It was developed as a result of the benefits observed from electro-acupuncture but, as its full name suggests, it works on the principle of stimulating the nerves.

**Method** An electrode is placed over segments of peripheral nerves or on acupoints. This is connected to a portable transistorised stimulator which delivers a high frequency, low intensity current, inducing a comfortable buzzing or tingling sensation which can be sustained for 30 minutes or more. One of the advantages of TENS is its portability. Patients can carry their own unit, like a transistor radio, and switch it on whenever pain relief is required.

**Result** The brief, intense stimulus of the electric current travels by the faster A nerve fibres (see page 18) which block or disrupt the pain messages travelling in the slower C fibres. This disruption can outlast the actual stimulation and relief may continue for some hours. Treatment can also induce a general feeling of well-being as well as reducing pain. TENS is often used as an alternative to long-term painkilling medication.

In 1975 Professor R. Melzack, one of the world's leading researchers into pain, reported having great success in the use of TENS: 75 per cent of peripheral nerve injuries, 60 per cent of phantom limb pain, and 62 per cent of shoulder and arm pain was relieved in experiments using TENS.

People who have had a heart pacemaker fitted should not use TENS as it can interfere with the action of the pacemaker.

## HOW IT CAN HELP

*TENS is useful for cases of prolonged, intractable pain, particularly the alleviation of persistent nerve pain. It is not, however, a substitute for proper medical treatment of the underlying causes of pain. Specific problems it can help include:*

► Sports injuries
► Lumbago
► Sciatica
► Phantom limb pain
► Shoulder and other joint pain
► Pain during childbirth

*ELECTRICAL PAIN RELIEF*
*In TENS treatment, electrodes that deliver electrical impulses are placed on the surface of the body or implanted under the skin.*

## ZERO BALANCING

Zero balancing combines methods designed to restore harmony to the body's energy fields with manipulative body-working techniques. It was developed by Dr Fritz Smith, an American osteopath and acupuncturist, who believed that working on the body's structure as well as its energy channels was the best way to stimulate the life force within the body and enhance the natural healing forces.

Unlike techniques such as acupuncture and shiatsu which concentrate on energy pathways near the surface of the body, zero balancing focuses on the energy channels that pass through the bones deep within the body. Practitioners believe this energy flow is most easily evaluated at the joints.

**Method** In a zero balancing session you will be asked to lie fully clothed on your back. The practitioner will examine the joints to discover their flexibility and range of movement, and then use sustained stretches and finger pressure to encourage the release of tension accumulated in the body. Zero balancing treatment works with the whole body, usually through the legs and the spine, and deals with each area of pain as it is uncovered. The treatment aims to create a feeling of deep relaxation, giving a person the opportunity to let go of stress, tension and pain.

### HOW IT CAN HELP

*Zero balancing is a gentle therapy which is particularly useful for:*

▶ Neck and back pain
▶ Stress-related disorders
▶ Migraine

**Result** The practitioner applies only gentle pressure and stretching movements that are well within the tolerance of the individual. This makes zero balancing particularly suitable for cases in which more vigorous procedures, such as massage, might be too painful. Many people report increased flexibility as well as relief from pain.

## THERAPEUTIC TOUCH

Therapeutic touch is the term used by Dr Dolores Krieger, Professor of Nursing at New York University, to describe the 'laying-on of hands' art of healing which she sought to revive by training nurses in the art. According to Krieger it does not require professional qualifications; almost anyone can use their hands to help if they are able to develop sensory skills.

**Method** In therapeutic touch, the hands do not usually touch the body but are held and moved an inch or two away from it. The treatment is founded on the belief that there is an energy field around the body which, with practice, it is possible to feel. The healer passes the palms of the hands over the body to detect areas of congestion and pain. The aim is to unblock congested areas in the body so that the energy can flow more smoothly.

**Result** Therapeutic touch can produce a deep relaxed feeling in the patient. Experiments with mice have shown that injuries heal faster when subjected to the energy of healing hands. You can learn to expand your own sense of energy and use it to help yourself, family and friends.

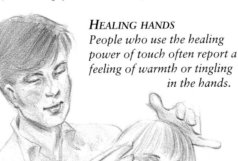

*HEALING HANDS*
*People who use the healing power of touch often report a feeling of warmth or tingling in the hands.*

### HOW IT CAN HELP

*Therapeutic touch can be used in any type of illness as an adjunct to other treatments, but in particular can give considerable relief in the painful stages of childbirth. It may also be useful for:*

▶ Neck and back pain
▶ Irritable bowel syndrome
▶ Chronic migraine

### FAITH HEALING

Healing has long been associated with religion, indeed Christianity is founded on belief in Christ's ability to heal. Faith healing is healing carried out in a religious setting. It usually takes place during a church service or prayer group meeting. Unlike other forms of healing, such as therapeutic touch, it is often carried out at a distance and need not involve touch or close contact.

# Natural Medicine

*Naturally occurring materials, such as plant extracts, can be used medicinally to alleviate pain. Herbs and plants contain a complex mixture of ingredients which act on the body's chemistry and physiology to relieve painful symptoms.*

## HOMEOPATHY

The basis of homeopathy is to give a very diluted dose of a substance which, if given to a fit person at full strength, would cause symptoms akin to the illness being treated.

**Method** Homeopathic medicines are derived from plant, animal and mineral compounds. A number of remedies are considered to have widespread application for painful disorders and can be obtained from any homeopathic pharmacy as well as chemists and healthfood shops.

However, a qualified practitioner of homeopathy will prescribe a more individualised remedy based on careful questioning about the nature of your pain and the various things that may influence its frequency and intensity. Pain resulting from cystitis, for example, might require different remedies in different patients, depending on various factors such as the degree and nature of the pain, whether the pain occurs before or after urination, and whether or not there is blood in the urine.

**Result** A homeopathic remedy that is well matched to your symptoms and other individual characteristics, such as your temperament or food preferences, will often be more effective in alleviating pain than a conventional painkiller. Homeopathic remedies do not cause any of the side effects associated with orthodox medication.

### HOW IT CAN HELP

*Homeopathy is effective for the treatment of a wide range of painful conditions including:*

► Digestive complaints
► Headaches and migraine
► Skin conditions such as eczema
► Premenstrual syndrome
► Joint ailments such as arthritis

### HOW HOMEOPATHY WORKS

Homeopathic medicines are produced by repeatedly diluting the original active component, a process known as potentisation. Each successive potency is signified by a number. The higher the number the more potent the remedy. Arnica 30, for example, is both more dilute and more therapeutically powerful than Arnica 6. Homeopathic remedies are usually taken in pill form.

A definitive explanation of how homeopathic medicines reduce inflammation or relieve pain has not been established. The amount of active ingredient in a remedy is so minute that it is not possible to detect any trace of it. Nevertheless, homeopathy has a proven track record and is widely accepted.

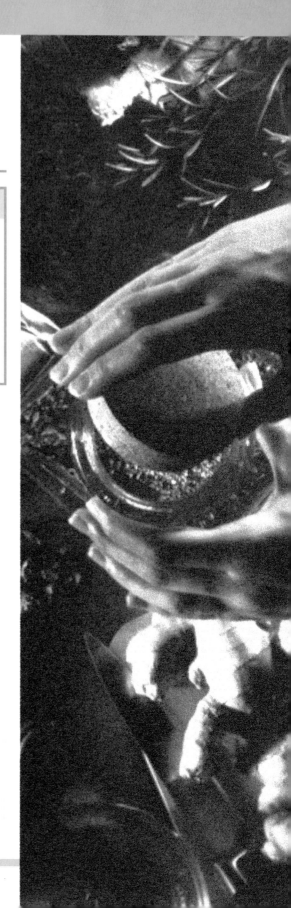

# HERBALISM

Throughout history plants have been used to treat painful disorders. Different traditions of herbal medicine have developed around the world, such as the Ayurvedic system in India, traditional Chinese medicine and the folklore remedies of the Native North Americans.

**Method** Modern medical herbalists and experts in pharmacognosy (the study of the chemical actions of plants) have identified many plant compounds which are used for pain control in different parts of the world. The active ingredients of medicinal plants are attracted to receptors on the cells of organs and tissues in the body. The ingredients fit into the receptors like jigsaw pieces and then initiate chemical changes that modify the function of the organ. Herbal remedies may be taken internally, for example in tablet form, or used externally, as a cream, lotion or ointment.

Herbs can relieve pain in a number of different ways, depending on their individual properties. For example, chilli peppers contain capsaicin which inhibits the action of the chemicals that relay pain messages to the brain. Marshmallow (*Althea officinalis*) has a high mucilage content, a sticky substance that helps to prevent irritation and ulceration of the digestive tract. Red sage (*Salvia officinalis*) relieves the pain of mouth ulcers and sore throats.

Medical herbalists usually prescribe a mixture of plant extracts that have complementary effects.

**Result** Herbal medicines have few side effects and are particularly suited to patients suffering from gastrointestinal disorders. As well as treating common illnesses, herbal medicines can relieve chronic conditions such as arthritis and migraine. They are also helpful in restoring general health and vitality.

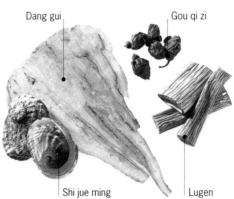

Dang gui    Gou qi zi

Shi jue ming    Lugen

***CHINESE HERBAL HEALING***
*Chinese herbalists have practised their art for centuries. Western science is currently researching the healing properties of a range of potent Chinese herbs.*

---

## HOW IT CAN HELP

*Herbalism is believed to be effective in a wide range of conditions. It is generally helpful at relieving pain or other symptoms associated with:*

► Skin disorders such as eczema

► Stress-related disorders

► Joint disorders, such as arthritis

► Digestive disorders, such as stomach ulcer and irritable bowel syndrome

► Respiratory disorders

► Sleep disorders, such as chronic insomnia

► Headaches and migraines

---

## SOME HERBS AND THEIR USES

The chart below shows a range of common pain problems that can be treated using herbs. It is important to treat herbs with respect; many have potent chemical components, and it is sensible to consult a qualified medical herbalist who can advise about the proper dosage.

| CONDITION | HERB | METHOD AND AIM |
|---|---|---|
| Sore throat, ulcers | Red sage *Salvia officinalis* | Use infusion or liquid extract as mouth rinse or gargle to soothe pain |
| Toothache | Oil of cloves | Apply oil of cloves on cotton wool to affected tooth |
|  | Camomile *Chamomilla* | Use camomile infusion as mouth rinse |
| Stomach ulcers | Liquorice *Glychyrriza glabra* Slippery elm *Ulmus fulva* | Drink liquid extracts of liquorice for pain Drink slippery elm powder in gruel to soothe inflamed mucous membranes |
| Colic, spasm, wind | Black hellebore *Helleborus niger*; Wild yam *Dioscorea villosa* (Ginger *Zingiber officinalis*) | Drink liquid extracts to relieve and prevent muscle spasms (Ginger assists action of other herbs – drink as tea) |
| Cystitis | Uva ursi *Arctostaphylos*; Marshmallow *Althaeaofficinalis* | Drink liquid extracts to soothe inflammation |
| Muscles and joints | Oil of wintergreen *Gaultheria procumbens*; Devil's claw *Harpagaphytum procumbens* | Massage oil of wintergreen into muscles and joints to soothe and relax Take devil's claw tablets |
| Migraine | Feverfew *Chrysanthemum parthenium* | Chew leaf or take tablets internally to ease pain |
| Neuralgia | Passionflower *Passiflora incarnata* | Drink liquid extracts to soothe pain |

# NATUROPATHY

Naturopathic medicine uses a wide range of approaches to restore and promote the body's healing powers. In many cases these can also be used to relieve pain. To achieve long-term health and well-being, naturopathy often requires a change in diet and other lifestyle factors in order to avoid the trigger factors that are causing the underlying condition.

The term 'naturopathy' is fairly recent, dating to the end of the 19th century. The principles upon which it is based, however, go back to the Greek physician Hippocrates (*c*.460-*c*.370 BC) who maintained that simple therapies such as diet could help the body to heal itself.

Modern naturopathy was pioneered by practitioners including Stanley Lief in the UK and Henry Lindlahr in the USA, who used measures such as hydrotherapy, osteopathy, massage and fasting to treat a wide range of medical disorders. Naturopaths were among the first to maintain that a healthy diet is one that is low in salt, saturated fats and processed foods.

**Method** Treatment might include physical measures, such as soft tissue massage, plus dietary and nutritional therapy and relaxation techniques. A naturopath may recommend various forms of hydrotherapy, such as hot and cold compresses, sprays and baths to stimulate the circulation to inflamed joints and other areas.

**Result** Naturopathy has proved beneficial in a range of conditions. For example, it can ease chronic disorders such as arthritis and reduce the need for painkillers. If you can incorporate elements of naturopathy into your lifestyle it can have a dramatic effect on your health.

## DIETARY AND NUTRITIONAL THERAPY

A major tool in naturopathic medicine is the use of dietary measures to support the body's self-healing mechanisms. For cases of inflammation or pain in the digestive or respiratory system, for example, a naturopath might recommend a 'juice fast' to cleanse the system, or a specially planned diet. The aim is to help the body direct its energies into resolving the underlying causes. A naturopath can also advise on foods to avoid in certain painful disorders. For example, coffee and chocolate can trigger migraine attacks in susceptible individuals. Naturopaths often recommend a combination of treatments, such as hot compresses together with a programme of dietary measures. Nutritional supplements may also be prescribed to modulate body chemistry in painful disorders, usually after carrying out tests to check for signs of mineral deficiencies.

## HOME HYDROTHERAPY FOR PAINFUL CONDITIONS

You can treat painful conditions by applying hot or cold water as a spray, a fomentation or a compress. To make a compress soak a large handkerchief or small towel in hot or cold water. Wring out, fold to size and place on painful part. Tie in place with a scarf or bandage.

| PAINFUL CONDITION | METHOD |
| --- | --- |
| Headache | Apply hot and cold fomentations to nape of neck – 2 minutes hot, 1 minute cold. Cold compresses to forehead – repeat frequently |
| Sinusitis | Apply hot and cold sprays or sponge to face – 2 minutes hot, 1 minute cold |
| Sore throat, pain in swallowing | Apply cold compress to throat for 2–3 hours or overnight |
| Painful cough | Apply hot and cold fomentations to chest – 3 minutes hot, 1 minute cold |
| Pain or colic | Apply hot compresses to abdomen – repeat frequently |
| Back, neck, or shoulder pains | Apply hot and cold fomentations to the painful area – 3 minutes hot, 1 minute cold, for 20–30 minutes once or twice daily |
| Knee, wrist, ankle injuries or pain | Apply cold compresses to the painful area for 1–2 hours or overnight |

# Mind Therapies

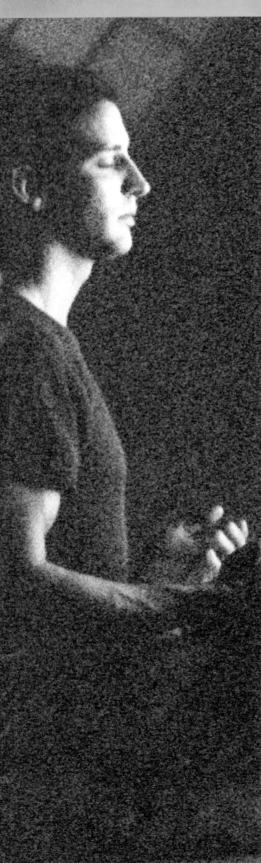

*Many therapies focus on calming the mind in order to reduce the perception of pain, or visualise it in a form that makes it easier to manage. Others attempt to resolve psychological conflicts and anxieties that are often associated with pain and its causes.*

## AUTOGENIC TRAINING

Autogenic training is a system of self hypnosis that uses special mental exercises to switch off the stress reactions of the body and replace them with restful, relaxed states. It can be used to relax the body prior to sleep, make the mind more receptive to change – for example, to stop bad habits – or to relieve painful illnesses. Autogenics literally means 'generated from within' and was first developed by neurologist Dr Johannes Schultz in the 1920s.

**Method**  Autogenics is based on the principle of 'passive concentration'. With practice, subjects develop a state of deep relaxation so they can give themselves positive suggestions designed, for example, to relieve tension, ease pain or stop smoking. There are six basic exercises that can be done anywhere, whether sitting or lying, to achieve a state of deep relaxation. These are taught over a series of sessions into which 'intention exercises' are gradually introduced. Autogenic exercises are tailored to the individual and may entail a period of concentration on the area causing the trouble. For example, you might be asked to imagine that your arms are heavy or your legs are hot. By concentrating on specific bodily sensations you can create a state of deep relaxation and learn to focus your attention inwards.

### HOW IT CAN HELP

*Autogenic training is effective for easing the pain from stress-related disorders. It can also relieve:*

▶ Migraine
▶ High blood pressure
▶ Fatigue
▶ Stomach disorders
▶ Period pains
▶ Menopausal pain

**Result**  It is believed that release of muscular tensions and even repressed emotions such as anger and grief may account for the effectiveness of autogenics. Some patients experience dramatic reactions to the therapy when repressed emotions are released.

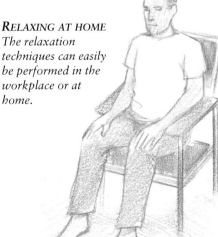

*RELAXING AT HOME
The relaxation techniques can easily be performed in the workplace or at home.*

## PSYCHOTHERAPY

Psychotherapy is a term which covers a wide range of approaches to the mental and emotional experiences of pain using talking and problem solving either on a personal or group therapy basis. Pain is the perception of a signal from the nervous system. Suffering is the negative reaction which complicates it. Psychotherapy offers help with these emotional components which can either be a result of the pain or can actually cause it.

**Method** Most psychological pain therapy is conducted by a trained therapist on a one-to-one basis. In group therapy people with common problems share their insights and experiences. Any psychotherapeutic help must be used in conjunction with proper attention to the physical causes of the pain.

Counselling varies from the guidance provided by religious leaders and priests to the more structured interviews with specially trained psychotherapists. In either case the opportunity to express fears and anxieties about pain and its causes can release some of the physical tensions associated with it.

**Result** The question of whether psychotherapy can make a significant difference to the management of pain is a popular subject for research. In a study reported in the British Journal of Medical Psychology (1959), therapy was used on a group of patients with musculoskeletal pain who also received physical therapy. A similar group of patients received physical therapy only.

Results showed that almost twice as many patients in the group receiving psychotherapy became pain-free compared with those in the control group.

### HOW IT CAN HELP

*Patients with painful disorders caused by some deeper underlying emotional or psychological problem can benefit from psychotherapy. Tension, stress, insomnia and phobias may all be caused by psychological problems. It can also be useful for physical ailments such as:*

▶ Cardiovascular disorders such as high blood pressure and angina

▶ Stomach disorders

▶ Bowel problems

▶ Headaches and migraine

### BEHAVIOURAL AND COGNITIVE PSYCHOTHERAPY

Faulty patterns of behaviour, such as using pain as a way of seeking attention, can often reinforce the likelihood of pain becoming chronic. The aim of behavioural psychotherapy is to break damaging thought cycles and reinforce positive behaviour patterns to cope with pain and reduce anxiety states. Behavioural therapy seeks to teach people coping mechanisms to help them to deal with their pain. Cognitive therapy is commonly used in pain management. The patient's thoughts, perceptions, and private interpretations can add to the distress of the physical symptoms. The major focus of cognitive therapy is to develop coping strategies by helping patients to plan and achieve goals for change.

## HYPNOTHERAPY

Hypnotherapy was developed in psychotherapy to provide faster results and a more accurate analysis of the patient's problems. Subjects suitable for hypnosis are placed in a trance which is said to provide the therapist with greater access to the patient's unconscious mind. In this way it is possible to uncover emotional blocks that cause psychological problems and prevent people from dealing with important life issues. In turn, obstacles to free expression can cause tension and stress-related problems such as headaches and chest pains.

**Method** While the patient is in a trance state the therapist will suggest positive mental images that help the patient to gain control over his or her physical condition. The practice of autosuggestion, or self-hypnosis, can also be taught so that patients can repeat the exercise at home. In some treatments, the therapist may explore the patient's subconscious mind in order to discover possible psychological causes of pain.

**Result** Hypnotism is effective at suppressing painful symptoms, but not necessarily the causes. With

### HOW IT CAN HELP

*Hypnotherapy is suitable for disorders with a strong psychological element, such as phobias, as well as psychosomatic disorders and stress-related conditions.*

hypnotherapy the relief from pain is usually temporary and the patient should consider other therapies to treat the cause. The main benefit for the patient may be the realisation that the mind can play a significant role in the perception of pain.

## VISUALISATION

Visualisation is based on the belief that the brain has a subconscious ability to heal, dating from primitive times in human development, that it cannot make use of on an intellectual level. By visualising positive images you can access this latent skill, for example, to modify nerve pathways that pass pain messages to the brain.

Using the close link between images and physical sensations, patients can be trained to exercise their imagination so that they can increase the input of positive impulses to the brain. It is suggested that these impulses can close the pain gate so that pain messages cannot be transmitted to the brain – a mechanism similar to that involved in transcutaneous electrical nerve stimulation or TENS.

**Method** Visualisation can be difficult to do alone at first so it is better to learn the techniques from an expert and then practise at home. The imagery that a therapist uses will depend on the nature of your pain.

For example, if you feel a hot, burning pain your therapist might choose cool images of water or ice flowing over the affected area, or you might visualise heat draining away like volcanic lava. Pain induced by cold or damp conditions may need the imagery of warmth and sunshine bathing the area.

**Result** Visualisation therapy for cancer patients was developed by Dr Karl Simonton. Simonton found that patients undergoing radiotherapy for cancer made better progress when they practised a form of visual imagery of the body's defences overcoming the tumours.

The therapy is most effective when the imagery chosen by the patient is something with which the individual can identify, such as a sports team beating its opponents. Visualisation is an integral part of many meditative and psychotherapeutic approaches. It is particularly effective when used in combination with breathing and relaxation exercises.

### HOW IT CAN HELP

*Visualisation is suitable for almost any kind of physical or emotional problem. It is particularly helpful for relieving pain caused by:*

▶ Cancer

▶ Angina

▶ Asthma

### PRACTISING VISUALISATION AT HOME

Visualisation can help you to manage pain. The following are two examples of the method but you will need to find images that work for you:

▶ *Imagine the pain is a fierce beast. Slowly build a wall around yourself to keep the beast away. Feel the pain ebb as the wall builds.*

▶ *See the pain as a shark. Surround yourself with dolphins to drive the sharks away. Feel the pain recede.*

## MEDITATION

Meditation embraces various contemplative practices, both religious and secular, as well as the more dynamic forms of ritual dance and movement. Vigorous dances designed to induce trance-like states are performed to rapid drum beats, often as a prelude to impressive feats. For example, fire walkers can walk or run over a pit of burning embers apparently without injuring their feet. The more accessible types of meditation are the contemplative forms used in spiritual retreats for Christian and Buddhist prayer and in disciplines with origins in Eastern mysticism such as yoga.

Whether dynamic or contemplative, meditation has been shown to lift the brain into the alpha rhythm state, that is, a state of relaxed awareness somewhere between full consciousness and sleep. In this state pain impulses are likely to be less intense. Meditation is often used as a prelude to more focused approaches such as visualisation.

**Method** You can meditate alone but may find it easier to get started if you practise with a group. Most people prefer a silent room, but if there is unavoidable background noise playing tapes of music or sounds of nature may create a more conducive atmosphere. Your meditation teacher may give you a mantra, a personal image on which to focus when meditating. As you concentrate on your breathing your mind will enter

### HOW IT CAN HELP

*Meditation is particularly effective at relieving chronic pain and discomfort caused by high levels of stress. It can also help to alleviate pain caused by:*

▶ High blood pressure

▶ Circulation problems

▶ Chest complaints such as asthma

▶ Migraine

the alpha rhythm state. Meditate for about 10 minutes at a time.

**Result** Meditation can provide relief from stress and, when practised on a regular basis, can lead to long-lasting effective pain relief.

# Relaxation Therapies

*Releasing muscular tensions and reducing mental tension are essential to the management of pain. There are methods using breathing and other techniques that can help to relieve pain and take advantage of the healing powers of relaxation.*

## PROGRESSIVE MUSCULAR RELAXATION

Rhythmical breathing to relax the muscles is the basis of most relaxation therapies. It is an integral part of yoga and other meditation techniques as well as of autogenic training. Many people use a meditation-like imagery to heighten the response but often the process of focusing on different areas of the body or particular muscle groups to relax them is enough to concentrate the mind.

**Method** As in all relaxation therapies it is important to find a comfortable position. Lying flat on your back with all joints free from pressure or restriction is usually the most suitable position. The nape of the neck and the knees can be supported with low pillows. Alternatively, relaxation therapy can be practised in a sitting

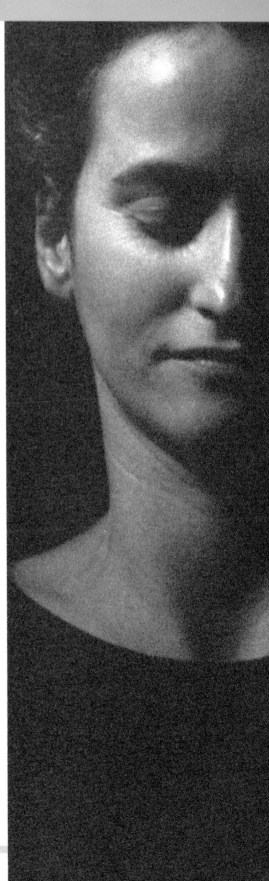

***RELEASE OF TENSION***
*Muscular relaxation techniques can be used to provide emergency stress relief.*

### HOW IT CAN HELP

*Progressive relaxation is useful as part of pain management programmes and stress relief. It has been found particularly effective in relieving chronic pains resulting from spinal injury.*

position, even at work, although it will not be possible to let go quite so completely.

It is best to learn relaxation techniques from a professional therapist and then practise at home. A therapist will usually start by encouraging you to establish a steady breathing rhythm. You will then be asked to focus the mind on one area of the body, such as the feet and legs for a few breaths, before moving up through the body a little at a time.

Some therapists use alternate tensing and relaxing techniques in which the muscle groups visualised are actively tightened and then released as the breath is exhaled. Patients are trained progressively in the use of such techniques until they are able to apply them on a daily basis at home or work.

**Result** Patients practising this method report a greater awareness of the body and more feeling of control.

# BIOFEEDBACK

Biofeedback is a system in which electronic instruments are used to give information about the body which might not otherwise be immediately obvious. The patient can use this information to control the body's activities in areas such as the brain and heart.

For some people the very process of progressive relaxation focusing on letting go of muscles is a contradiction. They may find it difficult to register the change in muscle tension and might tighten them again. Biofeedback instruments can help to overcome this by giving the user visual or audible information about the degree of tension in the body as the relaxation technique is practised.

**Method** The therapist will attach biofeedback instruments to the skin by electrodes, or alternatively you may be asked to hold the electrodes in your hands. Biofeedback instruments can work in a number of ways: some measure blood pressure or brain waves, others detect changes in pulse, temperature or the electrical resistance of the skin, which changes with sweating. These changes are usually indicated by a sound which changes in pitch or intensity, or by a needle or dial which rises or falls. As the person relaxes and tension is released, the sound reduces or the needle moves back. This is known as 'feedback' and gives the user a clear indication that they are achieving a more relaxed state. In time the patient will learn to achieve this state of relaxation without the aid of a biofeedback meter.

Biofeedback is valuable as a tool for learning general relaxation techniques and can be used in a more focused way in specific pain areas. For example, some biofeedback meters can be used to teach patients how to reduce their blood pressure, which is a vital aid in managing stress-related heart conditions.

**Result** Biofeedback has been found to be more effective in the management of head and neck pain than with back pain. Some studies have shown that over time biofeedback tends to be more useful for easing nervous tension than reducing muscle tension.

## HOW IT CAN HELP

*Biofeedback is particularly useful for achieving long-lasting relief from pain associated with nervous disorders such as fibromyalgia. It has also proved effective at reducing pain caused by stress, but is less effective in the treatment of depression-related ailments. If used in conjunction with yoga or other relaxation techniques, it can help to alleviate pain associated with:*

▶ High blood pressure

▶ Migraine

▶ Heart disease

▶ Childbirth

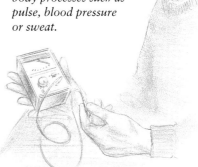

*BODY MONITORS
Biofeedback metres detect unconscious body processes such as pulse, blood pressure or sweat.*

# FLOTATION AND SENSORY DEPRIVATION

A flotation tank is an enclosed chamber in which the patient floats in water at skin temperature and in total darkness and silence. This sensory isolation tank gives complete freedom from external stimuli and enables the thoughts to focus inwards. It is said to help the user to gain greater control of the body and reduce blood pressure or pain.

**Method** The tank contains about 25–30 cm (10–12 in) of water at 34.2°C (93.5°F) in which Epsom salts and other minerals are dissolved to give buoyancy. You will be asked to take a shower before entering the tank. The therapist will give you earplugs to prevent irritation from the minerals and an inflatable pillow to support your head. You will then be left in darkness to float in the water for 15–30 minutes. If desired, soothing music tapes can be played to aid meditation and visualisation while in the tank.

**Result** An hour in a flotation tank is said to be the equivalent of 4 hours' sleep and can produce a state of deep relaxation. The method is an excellent stress reliever and the benefits can last up to four days.

## HOW IT CAN HELP

*Flotation is effective at inducing a deep feeling of relaxation and can help to minimise pain resulting from stress-related ailments. Recent research into the reasons for its effectiveness at relieving pain suggests that floating somehow stimulates the release of the body's natural painkillers, endorphins.*

▶ High blood pressure

▶ Heart disease

▶ Digestive ailments such as irritable bowel syndrome

▶ Migraine

▶ Sleep disorders, such as insomnia

# CHAPTER 5

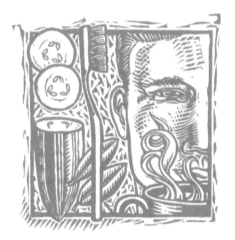

# HEAD AND THROAT PAIN

*Many of the painful conditions that affect the head, neck and throat can be successfully treated at home with natural therapies. Most ailments produce distinctive symptoms and with a knowledge of how these match the various types of pain affecting this area, you can learn to distinguish when you can deal with your pain safely at home and when you should consult a doctor.*

# HEADACHES

*Most headaches are not the result of a severe or life-threatening disorder, but occasionally they can act as a warning of a serious condition and should be investigated by a doctor.*

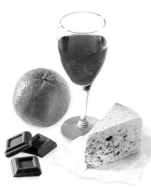

**MIGRAINE TRIGGERS**
*Eating cheese, chocolate or citrus fruits, or drinking red wine can trigger migraine attacks in some people. Other triggers could be waiting too long between meals, being overtired, or having too much or too little sleep. Stress and emotions such as worry and excitement have also been linked to migraine. Although depression can trigger migraines in susceptible individuals, research has shown that people who suffer from migraine are not as a group anxious or depressed.*

Pain in the head may have a variety of causes. It may result from muscle spasm, nervous tension, or an injury such as a trapped nerve caused by a crick in the neck. When the muscles in the head, face or neck go into spasm, blood vessels around them become over-constricted and then compensate for the constriction by dilating. Nerve fibres respond to the stretching of the blood vessels by sending pain messages to the brain.

The pain may be felt all over the head or it may occur in one part only. The sensation experienced can range from a superficial ache to a deep throbbing pain caused by blood rushing through the dilated arteries. By providing an accurate description of your headaches, including frequency and the pattern of occurrence, you can help your doctor to diagnose the problem and find the appropriate treatment. For example, a severe incapacitating headache that gets worse over time requires urgent medical attention, as it might indicate a dangerous brain disorder, such as a tumour. However, most headaches are a reaction to bad lifestyle traits such as irregular meals, poor posture or stress. Eyestrain, infection, an adverse reaction to particular foods, air conditioning, hangovers, lack of sleep, menstrual disorders, some prescribed drugs, and dental problems can also be responsible. In these cases the headache can be safely and successfully treated at home with simple painkillers, herbal medicine or relaxation. In the longer term a change in lifestyle is probably required to stop the headache recurring. More problematic are tension headaches and migraine, which while not life-threatening conditions, can disrupt a sufferer's life, causing persistent incapacitating pain, sometimes accompanied by nausea and sight disturbance.

## Migraines

Migraines are severe headaches which can last for anything from a few hours to a few days. They are caused by changes in the brain stem which cause the blood vessels around the brain to constrict. Blood flow then reduces to some parts of the brain. The constricted arteries start to dilate and stretch the sensitive nerve fibres around them which causes intense pain. Migraines almost always affect the same side of the head, the pain is intense and throbbing, and

---

### PROCESS OF A MIGRAINE

Migraines may be caused by tension, triggered by factors such as fatigue or stress. This sets off a sequence of events leading to pain. Many women are prone to migraines just prior to menstruation because of hormonal changes.

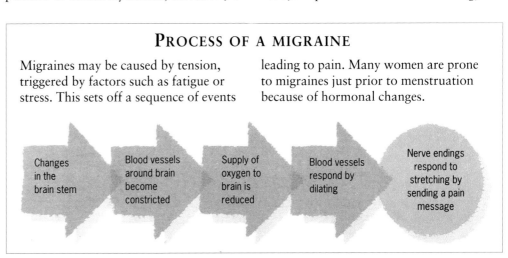

Changes in the brain stem → Blood vessels around brain become constricted → Supply of oxygen to brain is reduced → Blood vessels respond by dilating → Nerve endings respond to stretching by sending a pain message

is often associated with nausea, vomiting and hot flushes alternating with shivering spells. As the hours pass, the pounding pain becomes a steady ache and after a period of sleep it usually subsides.

Although migraine pain can be relieved with painkillers, the possibility of side effects make them less desirable. Strategies for managing migraines should focus more on preventing them occurring than the use of drugs. Migraines may be triggered by a number of factors including stress, food and changes in routine and environment. Note down what you eat and drink and any resulting headache in a pain diary (see page 44). This may help you to pinpoint a trigger factor, such as red wine or stress.

**Treatment** For many migraine sufferers, lying in a darkened room may be the only way of dealing with attacks. The herbal remedy feverfew (*Tanacetum parthenium*) has been shown to be effective in many cases. You can obtain feverfew tablets from health food shops or eat a few feverfew leaves chopped up in a sandwich. You can also drink it as an infusion, by pouring boiling water onto freshly picked feverfew leaves. Other possible treatments include

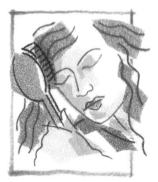

**HEADACHE REMEDY**

Whenever you feel a headache coming on, try 'brushing it away' using a moderately stiff hairbrush, or use your fingers to massage the scalp and relieve muscle tension:

■ *Starting above your eyebrow, draw the hairbrush over your scalp, back over the ear and down the back of the neck.*

■ *Go back to the top of the eyebrow, repeat the stroke again starting an inch to the right of the previous stroke.*

■ *Continue with the brush strokes until the head is covered.*

■ *Repeat every hour after pain relief to make sure the headache has really gone.*

## FIGHTING HEADACHES

Instead of using painkillers, there are several strategies that you can adopt to help prevent headaches recurring.

▶ *Transcutaneous electrical nerve stimulation (TENS). Research has shown that TENS (see page 83) can be effective at easing migraine pains. Equipment that sends out a mild electrical current to relax muscles painlessly is available for home use.*

▶ *Acupressure. For headaches with pain at the side of the head, use your thumbs to press underneath the base of your skull into the hollow areas on either side of the two vertical neck muscles. Tilt your head back with your eyes closed and continue pressing for 1–2 minutes as you breathe deeply.*

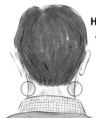

**Headache relief** You can apply acupressure to your neck yourself, or ask your partner or a friend to help you.

▶ *Taking exercise has the effect of dilating the blood vessels. This means that a brisk walk, a swim or bicycle ride can actually prevent blood vessels in the head from becoming constricted and sparking a headache. If you are already suffering a headache, exercise can help to return the blood vessels to their normal size and also stimulate the release of soothing endorphins. Regular walking, jogging or swimming can help to prevent the build up of tension in the neck and shoulders. However, always consult your doctor before starting a new exercise programme.*

Some can safely be practised at home; for others you will need to visit a complementary health practitioner.

▶ *Use your shower for hydrotherapy to relax your head and neck muscles. Turn the water temperature up as hot as is comfortable and direct the jet onto your back, neck, shoulders and scalp for at least five minutes. Massage the muscles at the same time. Once you feel relaxed, run cool water over the same areas for several minutes.*

**Hydrotherapy** You can practise hydrotherapy in your own home quite easily using a shower or shower attachment.

▶ *A 1996 study by the Royal Danish School of Pharmacy said that 81 per cent of migraine patients felt that reflexology had cured (16%) or helped (65%) their symptoms. Just under 20% said it enabled them to do without the medication they had been prescribed.*

▶ *Aromatherapy can prevent the onset of a headache. If you feel the symptoms coming on mix 1 or 2 drops of lavender oil with 5 drops of olive oil and massage in a circular motion across your temples, behind the ears and on the back of the neck.*

**Lavender baths** Ease tension by adding 3 drops each of lavender oil, marjoram and camomile to the bath.

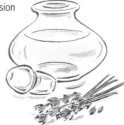

## TEETH CLENCHING

Some studies suggest that teeth clenching may be a causal factor in migraines. Prolonged periods of teeth clenching can trigger the release of substances called neuropeptides which can spark off a migraine. Current research suggests that if you can control your teeth clenching then you may be able to prevent migraine attacks.

▶ *When not chewing, aim to keep the teeth slightly apart.*

▶ *Try chewing sugar-free chewing gum to help to kick the habit.*

▶ *Prevent clenching during sleep by trying relaxation therapies before bedtime (see page 91).*

▶ *If you have a serious problem, your dentist can provide you with an appliance to prevent teeth clenching. This fits over the lower teeth and is worn at night.*

### WARNING
*Consult a doctor immediately if a headache comes on suddenly for no apparent reason and occurs with any of these symptoms:*
▶ *weakness, numbness or tingling in the limbs*
▶ *partial loss of consciousness*
▶ *a high fever*
▶ *skin rash*

Alexander Technique, massage, hypnotherapy, aromatherapy, naturopathy, acupuncture and acupressure.

▶ *see also manipulative, massage, energy, natural, mind, relaxation therapies*

### Temporomandibular disorder (TMD)
The temporomandibular joint connects the lower jaw bone with the temporal bone of the skull. When this joint and the muscles and ligaments that support it fail to function properly, it can result in pain in the head, jaw and face. Grinding the teeth together, which can result from tension in the jaw muscles, is one of the major causes of TMD. Typically patients complain of a stiff jaw, or difficulty in opening the mouth, tenderness over the jaw joint or noises from the joint such as clicking. Sufferers often mistakenly believe that the pain is coming from the ear or that the joint is damaged. However, TMD rarely leads to arthritis of the temporomandibular joint.
**Treatment** This depends on the severity of

the problem. Painkillers can be helpful, as can a hot compress applied to the painful area, jaw exercises, a soft diet, TENS (see page 83), and physiotherapy. Teeth covers can also be effective (see far left).

▶ *see also manipulative, movement, massage, energy, relaxation therapies*

### FACIAL PAIN
Pain in the face may be due to a variety of causes, such as injury or infection, but frequently it may occur for no apparent reason. Pain may be referred to the face from other parts of the body. The nerves supplying sensation to the face, including the sinuses, teeth, surface of the eyes, nose and skin, are all branches of a main nerve known as the trigeminal nerve. One main nerve supplies the right side and another supplies the left side. This means that if there is damage to one part of the face served by the trigeminal nerve it may be felt in another branch of the same nerve. For example, a patient may feel certain that the pain is from a tooth when in fact the pain may be referred to the tooth from a sinus problem on the same side.

In addition, an individual's psychological state can influence facial pain by mechanisms which are not fully understood. It is estimated that 10 per cent of patients who are depressed also suffer from facial pain.

### Sinus pain
In the skull and face there are 14 sinuses, or air-filled cavities in the bone. Infections, blockages, local growths or tumours can all

## SINUSES

The word 'sinus' is usually used to describe the air-filled cavity in the bones surrounding the nose (see right). These sinuses are lined with membranes which can become inflamed and cause pain. Known as sinusitis, this condition may be due to bacterial infection or in some cases a tooth abscess.

*THE SYMPTOMS OF SINUSITIS*
*Typical symptoms of sinusitis are a sensation of tightness in the affected area, which may develop into a throbbing pain, fever, a blocked nose and loss of sense of smell.*

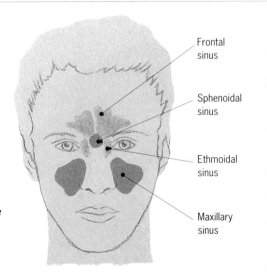

Frontal sinus

Sphenoidal sinus

Ethmoidal sinus

Maxillary sinus

give rise to problems with the sinuses. Most commonly, sinus pain is caused by an acute bacterial or viral infection such as the common cold. Infection spreads from the nose leading to inflammation of the membrane lining the sinus. Chronic sinus problems may be caused by small growths in the nose, smoking, irritant fumes and smells, and common respiratory and food allergies.

**Treatment** To open up the air passages and help to drain excessive mucus from the sinuses, try inhaling aromatherapy oils or steam. Place a few drops of eucalyptus oil with lemon onto a hankie and inhale deeply. Splashing or sponging the face and sinus areas with hot and cold water alternately (2 minutes hot and 1 minute cold) is effective at relieving pain.

If you feel a dull ache in your forehead, a simple acupressure technique may be helpful. Place the thumb and index finger of your left hand on either side of the bridge of the nose near the eyebrows. With the fingers and heel of your right hand grasp the muscles on either side of the spine at the back of the neck. Put pressure on all four points simultaneously while you breathe deeply for 1 minute.

If symptoms persist your doctor will usually prescribe antibiotics to clear the infection. In more severe cases surgery may be required to prevent further blockage.

▶ *see also manipulative, massage, energy, natural, relaxation therapies*

## Trigeminal neuralgia

Trigeminal neuralgia (TGN) is a painful disorder of the trigeminal nerve which usually affects people over the age of 40. Sufferers complain of a severe incapacitating pain which normally lasts for just a few seconds and is often described as lancinating, or like an electric shock. The pain can affect any area served by the trigeminal nerve but most commonly affects the mid face region.

**Treatment** Acupuncture and acupressure, may be effective at treating TGN. If you feel facial pain coming on, it may help to try pressing the end of your eyebrow near your nose with your finger. Applying hot and cold compresses to the area can help: apply a hot compress for 3 minutes followed by a cold compress for 1 minute, for a total of 20 minutes. As stress may be a contributing factor to the pain, relaxation therapies may be particularly useful. To relax the nervous

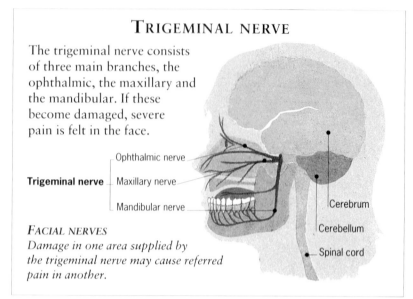

## TRIGEMINAL NERVE

The trigeminal nerve consists of three main branches, the ophthalmic, the maxillary and the mandibular. If these become damaged, severe pain is felt in the face.

**Trigeminal nerve** — Ophthalmic nerve / Maxillary nerve / Mandibular nerve — Cerebrum, Cerebellum, Spinal cord

*FACIAL NERVES*
*Damage in one area supplied by the trigeminal nerve may cause referred pain in another.*

system, add 2 drops each of essential oil of lavender and basil to steam inhalations, baths and massage oils. Some sufferers have found relief by increasing their intake – up to 600 mg daily – of vitamins $B_1$, $B_6$ and $B_{12}$ which can help to improve nerve function.

The conventional treatment for trigeminal neuralgia is carbamazepine. If this drug fails to control the pain or causes serious side-effects surgery is usually carried out.

▶ *see also massage, energy, natural therapies*

## Atypical facial pain

Atypical facial pain (AFP) is a condition that most commonly affects middle-aged women. Sufferers usually complain of constant pain over a bony area on one side of the face. If you suffer from this type of pain, it is essential to consult a doctor so that he or she can perform tests to rule out the possibility of serious bone or sinus disease.

**Treatment** As depression may contribute to AFP, meditation and hypnotherapy may help to limit the recurrence of attacks. Therapies that work on the body's energy pathways, such as shiatsu, acupuncture, acupressure and TENS may also be effective. Conventional treatment also addresses the emotional aspect of the pain and so antidepressants are commonly prescribed for AFP. However, a lower dosage is prescribed than that for patients suffering clinical depression. Treatment is generally successful, although the drugs may be prescribed over months or even years and must be taken daily throughout this period.

▶ *see also massage, mind, relaxation therapies*

# EAR, MOUTH AND THROAT PAIN

*Problems with the ear, mouth and throat can usually be diagnosed quickly and successfully treated, but dental treatment or special investigation may sometimes be necessary.*

The ears, mouth and throat are among the most sensitive organs in the body and consequently are susceptible to a variety of disorders. Most of the commonest conditions are easily treated at home.

### EARACHE

Earache is an extremely common condition, particularly in children. The most common cause is infection, which can affect all three sections of the ear: the outer ear, the middle ear and the inner ear. Occasionally, pain may feel as if it is in the ear when in reality it results from problems in neighbouring areas such as the neck or throat, which are served by the same nerves as the ear.

## Problems of the outer ear

A sore and inflamed ear, with scaly skin around it, are generally signs of problems of the outer ear. You may also experience a slight watery discharge. These symptoms may indicate a common condition, otitis externa, which is essentially a skin problem. You may feel a strong desire to poke the ear with anything that might be available, such as a matchstick or pen, but this could damage the eardrum. Boils in the ear canal can cause considerable discomfort and will require medical attention. Excessive ear wax, a secretion produced by glands in the outer ear, can also cause irritation.

**Treatment** Warm almond oil applied with a cotton bud can relieve minor skin problems affecting the outer ear and also soften ear wax so it can be removed more easily. However, if problems persist you should consult a doctor because it may be necessary to clean the ear canal. This should not be attempted at home as the use of cotton buds or other implements may simply push the ear wax deeper into the canal.

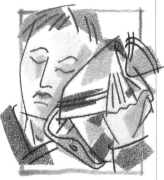

## EARACHE ANTIDOTES

For immediate relief from earache, try:

■ *Two drops of essential oil of St John's wort in the affected ear.*

■ *Hold a warm hot-water bottle wrapped in a towel to the ear.*

■ *In the longer term, eliminating dairy products from your diet can help to prevent mucus from obstructing the eustachian tube. Instead of cow's milk or cheese, try soya or goat's milk and cheese.*

---

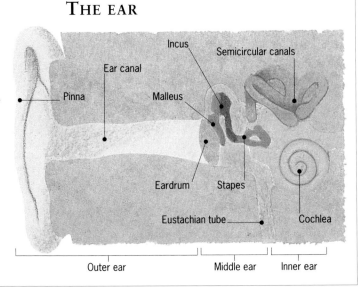

## THE EAR

The most common disorders of the ear occur in the middle ear, which includes the eardrum, malleus, incus, stapes and eustachian tube. In most cases earache is due to infection.

*EAR CARE*
*The ears are delicate organs vital for balance and hearing. They should be safeguarded from excessive noise.*

Pinna · Ear canal · Incus · Semicircular canals · Malleus · Eardrum · Stapes · Eustachian tube · Cochlea

Outer ear · Middle ear · Inner ear

## Problems of the middle ear

If earache is associated with other symptoms such as impaired hearing, the problem is usually in the middle ear. This type of earache is often experienced by adults when flying (see right). Pain in the middle ear is common in children because the eustachian tube which regulates air pressure in the middle ear is shorter in infants, so infections can easily spread from the throat. There may be inflammation and a build-up of fluid in the middle ear, a condition called otitis media. Pressure can build up behind the eardrum, causing severe earache. In some cases the eardrum perforates, relieving the pressure and easing the pain. The eardrum soon heals and there is usually no lasting damage. **Treatment** Otitis media is usually treated with antibiotics. In cases of chronic otitis media, a small tube or 'grommet' may be inserted into the eardrum to allow fluid to escape and prevent a build-up of pressure.

## Problems of the inner ear

If you experience dizziness or any disturbance of balance, you should consult your doctor immediately as it could indicate a serious disorder of the inner ear such as Ménière's disease that can lead to deafness.

### MOUTH PAIN

The mouth has a complex structure, reflecting its important role in eating, drinking and speaking. As many diseases caused by bacteria, viruses or fungi can be transmitted orally it is very vulnerable to infection.

## Mouth ulcers

A mouth ulcer is a break in the lining of the mouth. Most common are aphthous (pronounced ap-thus) ulcers which occur alone or in groups on the inside of the lips, the cheeks or underneath the tongue. Affecting about 1 in 5 of the adult population, minor aphthous ulcers are recurrent and heal in about two weeks. The commonest cause of these ulcers is a deficiency in minerals and vitamins such as iron, vitamin $B_{12}$ and folic acid. Stopping smoking often leads to aphthous ulcers for reasons which are unclear. Biting the lip or tongue can also trigger aphthous ulcers in susceptible individuals. **Treatment** Research has shown that 40 per cent of aphthous ulcer patients have low levels of vitamin $B_1$ and $B_6$. If you suffer from aphthous ulcers, taking $B_1$ and $B_6$

supplements for four weeks may help to prevent further outbreaks. The recommended dose for an adult is 300mg of vitamin $B_1$ and 50mg of vitamin $B_6$ three times a day.

If you continue to suffer from aphthous ulcers but your blood levels of iron, vitamin $B_{12}$ and folic acid are normal, and you don't respond to vitamin $B_1$ and $B_6$ therapy, it is worth considering other factors such as food allergy. The main food substances which trigger aphthous ulcers are benzoates (food additives), cinnamon and chocolate. Benzoates, which are listed on food labels with the code numbers E210-219, are principally found in fizzy drinks, particularly diet drinks. (Ordinary and diet 7-Up contain no benzoates.) Cinnamon is found in certain curries, cakes, sweets and tartar control toothpaste. If products containing these substances are avoided, aphthous ulcers tend to heal quickly and not recur.

▶ *see also energy, natural therapies*

## Cold sores

Cold sores, or herpes labialis, are small blisters which form around the mouth. They are caused by a herpes virus often acquired in childhood. The initial infection can produce widespread mouth and lip ulcers. After the first outbreak the virus 'hides' in the nerves that supply the lips and facial region but is sometimes reactivated causing cold sores. They can be triggered by sunlight, colds, menstruation, trauma, stress, or for no apparent reason. Cold sores are highly infectious when the blisters are moist and sufferers can transfer the virus to other sites on their own body, such as the nailbed or the eyes. The virus can also be transmitted to other people by direct contact such as during kissing or oral sex.

**Treatment** The conventional treatment for cold sores is with ointment such as acyclovir cream, which effectively reduces the severity and duration of an attack. Geranium oil applied to cold sores every hour can help to relieve pain and aid healing. The antiseptic effect of lemon juice rubbed on the lips when you feel a cold sore coming on may also inhibit the virus. Note that ointments and creams are far more effective if they are applied as soon as the first tingle of a developing cold sore is experienced. It is also important to apply the cream to a much larger area than the tingle seems to cover. A good antiseptic to apply to the lips at this

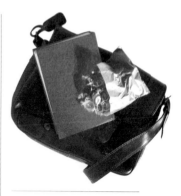

### EASING AEROPLANE EARACHE

Both adults and children frequently experience earache during or after an aeroplane flight. This is brought on by the difference in air pressure between the cabin and the middle ear. The following may help to equalise the air pressure in your ear:

▶ *Take a deep breath, pinch your nose shut, close your mouth and try to breathe out but don't do so. Swallow at the same time.*

▶ *Suck a sweet or chew gum on take off and landing to encourage vigorous swallowing.*

▶ *If flying with a baby, breast or bottle feed the infant during take off and landing – the sucking action will help to equalise air pressure in the baby's ear.*

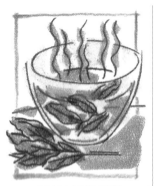

**SORE THROAT ANTIDOTES**

To ease the pain caused by a sore throat, rest your voice and try any of the following:

■ *Gargle with red sage – infuse 2 teaspoons of leaves in 200 ml (⅓ pint) boiling water for 10 minutes – for 10 minutes twice daily.*

■ *Eat a chicken broth, rich in zinc, to top up your fluids and nutrients and assist your immune system in the healing process.*

■ *Mix 2 drops each of eucalyptus and peppermint oils with 2 teaspoons of carrier oil and apply to the chest and throat area.*

time is distilled witch hazel and a tincture of myrrh combined in equal quantities. To prevent the recurrence of cold sores, it may help to increase your intake of iron-rich foods such as spinach, pulses and broccoli as research has shown that many cold sore sufferers have an iron deficiency.

▶ *see also massage, energy therapies*

## SORE THROATS

Sore throats are common in both adults and children. They may be the first symptom of the onset of a common cold, flu and laryngitis, as well as many childhood illnesses such as chickenpox and mumps. However, in most cases the condition lasts only a few days and provided the sufferer has an adequate fluid intake, and no other symptoms emerge, it is usually not serious enough to warrant a visit to a doctor.

**Treatment** Try gargling with a soluble painkiller such as aspirin or paracetamol before swallowing it. Alternatively gargling with salt or a herbal mixture such as sage or thyme (see left) or 2 drops of essential oil of lemon and sandalwood in warm water helps to soothe the throat.

### Acute tonsillitis

Tonsillitis is an inflammation of the tonsils due to infection. This highly infectious condition can be distinguished from a general sore throat by looking at the back of the throat – in acute tonsillitis the throat will be inflamed and there will be white spots on the tonsils. In addition, acute tonsillitis is generally more debilitating because it also causes fever symptoms.

**Treatment** If acute tonsillitis is suspected, it is probably best to stay at home and rest. Gargling a warm infusion of soluble aspirin or sage can help. Antibiotics can shorten the duration and severity of tonsillitis but are by no means necessary as the condition usually clears up in a few days.

### TOOTH AND GUM PAIN

The gums are the soft tissue surrounding the teeth which, when healthy, should be firm and pink or brown. Gum disease causes the gum tissue to become inflamed and you may see blood on your toothbrush or on an apple you've bitten into.

## Infected gums

The gums are particularly susceptible to infections such as gingivitis, periodontitis and the more unusual acute necrotising gingivitis (ANUG) which affects the lower front teeth. These conditions are caused by bacteria, but the bacteria responsible are different from those that cause tooth decay. Incomplete brushing allows plaque and tartar to build up on the teeth. Also known as calculus, tartar is formed when existing plaque becomes calcified from minerals in the saliva. This causes the gum around the margin of the tooth to become inflamed and reduces the periodontal ligament, which anchors the tooth in the bone, so that the gum bleeds easily on brushing or flossing.

You must attend to gum problems immediately. If you don't, inflammation around the tooth will increase and more of the periodontal ligament will be lost. Eventually the bony support of the tooth will be eroded, leading to bad breath and tooth loss. This process, which takes many years, is painless and occurs even when gums look healthy.

**Treatment** A healthy diet, including plenty of iron (good sources are wholemeal bread and dried apricots), careful brushing of the teeth twice a day, flossing at least once a day and regular visits to the dentist or hygienist all help to promote healthy gums. Other measures include mouthwashes and tartar control toothpaste. Ideally, an adult with natural teeth should have a dental check-up and polish every six months.

For bleeding and inflamed gums, rinse your mouth for one minute with several mouthfuls of a 0.1 per cent solution of folic acid and then swallow. Folic acid tablets taken daily may be effective in more severe

---

## TEETH AND GUMS

The most sensitive part of the tooth is the pulp which contains nerves and blood vessels. It is protected by dentine and enamel. The periodontal ligament acts as a shock absorber, cushioning the teeth and jaw when food is chewed.

*TEETH CARE*
*Regular dental check-ups help to control plaque build-up and warn of gum problems.*

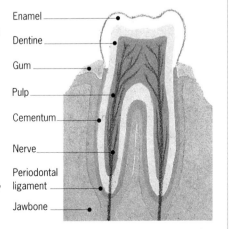

Enamel
Dentine
Gum
Pulp
Cementum
Nerve
Periodontal ligament
Jawbone

## TOOTH DECAY

If the protective enamel coating of a tooth becomes weakened, it may become eroded. Cavities soon start to form and sweet or very hot or cold food and drink then have access to the inner dentine layer and can cause sharp pain. Bacteria enter the cavities, leading to an infection that can spread through the tooth.

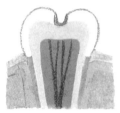 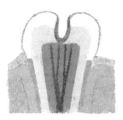 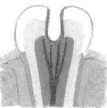 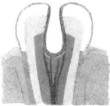

**Acids** formed from the breakdown of food wear away areas of enamel

**Bacteria** enter cavities in the enamel and attack the underlying dentine

**Decay** spreads to the pulp at the centre of the tooth, causing toothache

**The pulp** is destroyed and the tooth dies, and infection may spread. Pain subsides

### PREVENTING TOOTH DECAY

You can help to prevent painful tooth problems with a few simple measures:

▶ *Limit sugar intake. The more frequent the sugar intake, the more frequently teeth are exposed to an acid environment.*

▶ *Brush teeth twice daily and use floss every day.*

▶ *Visit your dentist or hygienist for a check-up every six months.*

▶ *Fluoride supplements, treatments and toothpastes can toughen a tooth against acid attack by strengthening the mineral composition of the enamel. To prevent the risk of fluorosis – a dark mottling of the teeth – children should not use more than a pea-sized amount of toothpaste and fluoride tablets should not be taken without consulting your dentist.*

cases. Some people report that chewing cardomom seeds helps to keep gums healthy. ANUG is usually treated with chlorhexidine mouthwash and antibiotics.

▶ *see also massage, energy, natural therapies*

### Teeth problems

The main problem affecting teeth is decay caused by plaque – food, saliva and bacteria – which coats the teeth and turns sugars into acids. These acids bleach minerals from the teeth in a process called demineralisation. This initially leaves the outer surface of the tooth enamel intact but shows up as a white spot. At this stage, the tooth decay is painless. If the process continues, however, bacteria can invade the inner dentine layer and pain will start to develop.

If the condition is left untreated, the infected pulp will die, often leading to a dental abscess. This is a pus-filled sac that forms as infection spreads into the tissue around the root of the tooth. This causes constant toothache, the surrounding gum becomes red, swollen and tender, and biting and chewing are very painful. The abscess may spread through the tissues and into the jaw bone, causing inflammation and swelling in the face and neck. A serious infection can destroy bone around the root area.

**Treatment** Minor tooth decay can be treated by a simple dental filling. However, if the pulp of a tooth is affected, as in irreversible pulpitis, it must be removed and the tooth filled. If an abscess forms, your dentist may prescribe antibiotics to treat the infection. The dentist will need to drain the abscess to release the build-up of pus, before extracting the tooth. After a tooth has been removed, blood fills the tooth socket and clots; over a period of several weeks the area will heal up completely.

Occasionally, and particularly in the case of lower molar teeth, the blood clot does not form properly, causing a painful condition known as dry socket. This can be relieved with a zinc oxide dressing from the dentist. Alternatively, for any tooth pain, oil of cloves applied to the painful area provides short-term relief.

▶ *see also massage, energy, natural therapies*

### Other causes of toothache

Your dentist may take radiographs of the teeth, jaws and sinuses to eliminate other causes of pain such as sinusitis (see page 96). Sinusitis may cause toothache because the roots of the upper teeth project into the maxillary sinuses and irritation of the lining of the sinuses can stimulate the nerves in the teeth and mimic toothache. This condition is usually easy to distinguish from the pain associated with tooth decay because it affects several teeth at the same time.

Toothache may also be due to receding gums which expose the layer that covers the root, called the cementum. Toothbrushing can wear away the cementum, exposing the underlying dentine and making the tooth susceptible to pulpitis. Receding gums may be treated by sealing off the dentine with dental adhesive. Rarely, toothache may indicate a problem with the facial bones such as misalignment of the jaw.

# THE EYES

*The eye is a complex organ that converts images into nerve signals and sends them to the brain for analysis. Most pain in the eyes is minor, but in serious cases the sight may be at risk.*

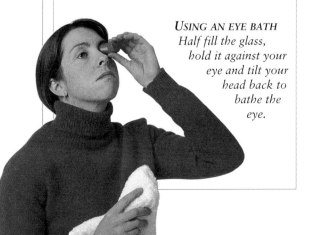

## TREATING YOUR EYES

To ease tired aching eyes, take time to give them a special treat:

■ *For sore eyes, mix some juice from an aloe vera plant with warm water and bathe the eyes.*

■ *For swollen, baggy eyes, place cold used tea bags or cucumber slices over each eye.*

■ *For dry tired eyes, boil a pint of water with a pinch of baking soda, leave to cool, then use the solution to bathe the eyes.*

Minor disorders of the eye and the surrounding area, such as blepharitis, a scaly condition of the eyelid, can be safely treated at home, either with conventional or complementary methods. More serious conditions must be treated by professionals. Although painful eye problems are usually accompanied by loss of vision, many serious progressive conditions are painless making self-diagnosis difficult. You can help to avoid serious eye problems by reporting the onset of any symptoms promptly to your doctor or optician. You should rest your eye muscles at regular intervals during concentrated use and wear protective eye gear when doing potentially harmful activities such as DIY.

### Preventing eyestrain

If your work involves concentrated use of the eyes, such as for reading or using a computer, rest your eye muscles every half hour. You can do this by focusing on an object in the distance. Without taking your eyes off the object, gently sway from side to side.

If you wear contact lens, keep your lens containers as clean as possible to prevent infection (using distilled water or boiled tap water). Eat plenty of green and yellow vegetables for vitamin A, the essential vitamin for the eyes. Wear optical quality sunglasses in the snow and in bright sunlight to avoid damage from ultra violet light.

### Chronic glaucoma

Chronic glaucoma is a potentially blinding condition which is completely treatable if diagnosed early. Affecting 1 in 200 of the population over the age of 40, this common condition is caused by damage to nerve fibres from excessive pressure of the fluid in the eye. Although glaucoma is often painless in the early stages, if it is not detected it can cause severe pain in and around the eye and loss of vision in the later stages. The condition is detected by measuring the eye pressure and should be done as part of a routine eye test by the optician. You should see an optician immediately if you experience unfamiliar pain in the eyes, or loss of peripheral vision, or blurring of vision.

**Treatment** Most forms of glaucoma can be controlled by taking regular medication, usually eye drops, but sometimes tablets or capsules. In some cases, minor eye surgery is needed to reduce fluid pressure in the eye.

---

### MAKING AN EYE BATH

To make a soothing eye bath, add 1 teaspoon of eyebright to a teacup of boiling water. Cover and leave to cool, then strain through coffee filter paper and use the solution to bathe the eyes.

*USING AN EYE BATH*
*Half fill the glass, hold it against your eye and tilt your head back to bathe the eye.*

---

### CAUTION
*If you experience any of the following symptoms consult a doctor: redness of the eye, sudden loss of vision, black spots that obstruct vision, flashing lights, double vision, excessive watering of an eye together with pain.*

# CHAPTER 6

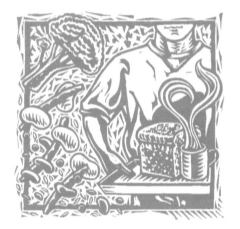

# CHEST AND ABDOMINAL PAIN

*From heartburn to heart attack, from indigestion
to appendicitis, pain may occur in the chest and in
the abdomen for reasons that vary hugely in severity.
A knowledge of the different kinds of pain and the
underlying causes will help you to decide whether
your symptoms indicate a minor problem – as
is most likely – or a serious condition which
requires urgent medical investigation.*

# CHEST PAIN

*Many people panic unnecessarily when they experience chest pain. Very often problems are minor and easily treated. Some kinds of chest pain, however, require careful monitoring.*

## PREVENTING HEARTBURN

Heartburn is often associated with overeating or with rich and spicy foods. By paying careful attention to your diet and general health you can help to prevent heartburn.

▶ *Eat small meals.*

▶ *Avoid fatty foods, including those with 'hidden' fat such as pastry.*

▶ *Lose weight if you are overweight.*

▶ *Wear loose clothing avoiding tight belts.*

▶ *Relax before and after eating.*

▶ *If you get heartburn at night in bed, raise the head end of the bed by a few inches to elevate you.*

▶ *Avoid stooping at the waist.*

▶ *Stop smoking as smoking reduces the effectiveness of the cardiac sphincter (see right).*

Many common chest complaints are caused by minor problems such as a strained muscle or heartburn. However, in some cases chest pain may indicate a condition which needs urgent medical investigation, such as a heart attack. Several causes of chest pain are outlined below, with self-help treatments and guidance on when to seek medical advice.

## Heartburn

Heartburn is a common complaint and is usually described as a burning sensation behind the sternum, or breast bone. It is caused by a backflow of acids from the stomach into the gullet, or oesophagus, the tube which carries food to the stomach. This usually occurs because of a failure of a ring of muscle called the cardiac sphincter which separates the oesophagus from the stomach. When functioning normally, this muscle opens to allow food through and then closes to keep it inside the stomach

(see below). Heartburn is often brought on by overeating, or by eating chocolate, spicy food, and fatty foods which relax the sphincter. Other foods such as coffee, cola and beer can increase the pain of heartburn because they increase the acidity of stomach juices. Changing position, such as lying down or bending over, can all precipitate the pain. Mild infrequent heartburn does not usually require medical investigation, but if symptoms get worse or cannot be controlled by simple measures, you should seek medical help as this may indicate a more serious condition such as oesophagitis (inflammation of the oesophagus).

**Treatment** During an attack of heartburn, sit up. If it's a bad attack at night you may find it more comfortable to sleep in a chair. Antacids are usually effective and drinking milk can be helpful. Hot compresses placed over the stomach can improve the blood supply in the area and relax the muscles. Conventional over-the-counter medicines,

## WHY HEARTBURN 'BURNS'

The cardiac sphincter muscle connects the oesophagus with the stomach. If this muscle fails to close properly, stomach acids can flow back into the oesophagus. Here, the acids cause the typical burning pain associated with heartburn as the lining of the oesophagus is not as well protected as the stomach lining.

*THE STOMACH'S 'VALVE'*
*The cardiac sphincter muscle stops the contents of the stomach flowing back into the oesophagus.*

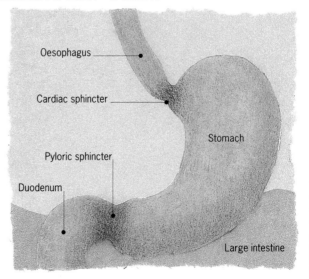

Oesophagus

Cardiac sphincter

Stomach

Pyloric sphincter

Duodenum

Large intestine

including antacids to neutralise the stomach acids, provide effective relief. Herbalists may recommend an infusion of slippery elm tablets or marshmallow root. Homeopathic remedies are available, and acupuncture and acupressure may also be helpful.

▶ *see also massage, energy, natural therapies*

## Painful cough

A cough is a reflex action to clear irritants or blockages in the breathing passages or respiratory tract. Burning coughs felt behind the breast bone can be caused by tracheitis, inflammation of the windpipe, or trachea. Hoarse coughing accompanied by pain in the throat may indicate laryngitis, or inflammation of the larynx. A sharp pain in the ribs when coughing or taking a deep breath, may indicate pleurisy – inflammation of the lining of the lung. This requires immediate medical attention.

**Treatment** Conventionally, a cough can be treated with painkillers, such as paracetamol, and cough medicines. Homeopathic remedies for coughs are also available. - Essential oils such as eucalyptus, myrrh, sandalwood or frankincense can be added to a bowl of hot water and inhaled, or massaged onto your chest and back, to help to ease the pain. Sprinkling a few drops of myrrh on the pillow aids breathing at night.

▶ *see also massage, energy, natural therapies*

## Chest infection/Bronchitis

An acute chest infection usually follows a cold and is characterised by a cough with phlegm. The cells lining the respiratory tract produce the phlegm to help entrap the irritant so it can be coughed out. If you have a chest infection you may also experience shortness of breath and the cough can be painful. When coughing, pain is usually felt in the windpipe, or in the muscles between the ribs. A chronic cough or one that produces green or yellow phlegm should be reported to a doctor as this may indicate infection requiring antibiotic treatment.

**Treatment** The best way to relieve the pain from a chest infection is to encourage the removal of phlegm from the body rather than suppress it with over-the-counter cough remedies. To help keep phlegm loose during a chest infection drink at least 2 litres of fluids a day (avoid milk, however, as this encourages mucus build-up) and take plenty of rest. Avoid cold air, smoke and fog, and smokers should try to give up cigarettes. Steam inhalation can be useful for bringing up phlegm. Eating garlic on a regular basis is a proven preventative which can help to reduce the risk of catching a chest infection.

▶ *see also massage, energy, natural therapies*

## Angina

Angina is the pain which people experience when the blood supply to the heart is impaired. It is commonly described as a tight constriction or pressure across the centre of the chest, and can often be felt in the left arm, neck or jaw. During an attack you may feel short of breath, nauseous, dizzy and sweaty. Angina can be provoked by a heavy meal, exercise, cold weather or stress. If you experience a new pain, or if the pain persists despite using prescription medication, or if the pain starts without any obvious factors triggering it, you should consult your doctor at once.

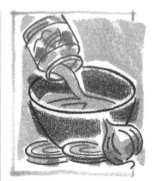

**SOOTHING COUGHS**

You can make simple cough remedies from natural ingredients in your kitchen.

■ *To make a cough mixture, slice an onion into a deep bowl, cover it in honey, and leave to stand overnight. Strain the mixture well into a clean bottle or jar and take one teaspoon up to five times a day.*

■ *For a dry irritating cough, use an infusion of fresh or dried marshmallow leaves.*

■ *If you're suffering from excessive phlegm, try this tea. Take 5g of ginger powder, a pinch of clove powder and a pinch of cinnamon powder. Place the ingredients in a mug, pour boiling water over and stir well.*

## TREATING CHEST INFECTIONS

Although chest infections are rarely contagious, they can cause considerable discomfort. There are several steps you can take at home to relieve the aching pain under the breast bone. However, if the chest infection is accompanied by sinus problems, earache or pneumonia, medical treatment is necessary.

**DRINK MORE LIQUIDS**
*Drinking extra liquid keeps the phlegm more fluid.*

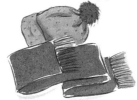

**KEEP WARM AND REST**
*Keeping warm and resting will help the body to recover.*

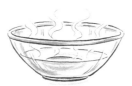

**ADD MOISTURE TO THE AIR**
*Extra humidity will help to bring the phlegm up and out.*

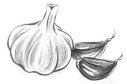

**EAT GARLIC**
*Garlic can help to prevent further chest infections.*

## PREVENTING ANGINA

You can take steps to prevent the onset of angina by watching your diet carefully and learning to listen to your body:

▶ *Stop smoking – the risk of dying from heart disease will be significantly reduced by limiting further hardening of the arteries by nicotine and carbon monoxide.*

▶ *Maintain your weight at a level appropriate for your height and age. This will help to keep blood pressure lower and reduce strain on the heart.*

▶ *Reduce or eliminate animal fats and salt in your diet and incorporate larger amounts of fibre, fish and garlic. This will also reduce the risk of hardening of the arteries.*

▶ *Manage stress with mind therapies (see page 88) such as meditation and autogenic training, and with gentle exercise.*

*HAWTHORN TEA*
*Try an infusion of 2 teaspoons of hawthorn berries steeped in a cup of hot water for 20 minutes – it is known to improve heart function.*

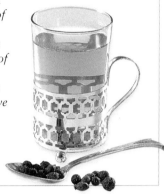

**Treatment** Patients suffering from angina are usually prescribed drugs and advised to give up smoking, to take regular exercise and take steps to manage any stress more efficiently. Naturopaths can offer advice on dietary management and nutritional supplements such as magnesium and vitamin E. Many homeopathic remedies may relieve the symptoms and are sometimes used in conjunction with conventional treatments. However, if you observe any changes in the frequency or intensity of your angina pain, consult a doctor as soon as possible.

▶ *see also movement, mind, relaxation therapies*

*EXERCISE AND ANGINA*
*Regular gentle exercise such as walking can be of enormous benefit to angina sufferers. Exercise strengthens the heart and improves circulation. Start gently and increase the amount of exercise gradually.*

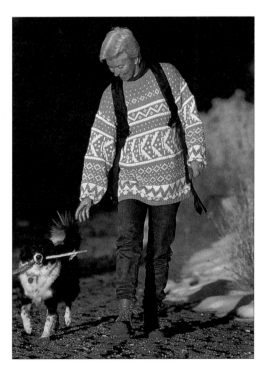

## Heart attack

A heart attack is a life-threatening condition but with prompt medical attention and sensible changes to lifestyle, many heart attack victims recover to lead a long and healthy life. A heart attack is caused by an interruption of the blood supply to the heart muscle, usually because of a blockage such as a blood clot, or thrombus, in an artery.

Heart attack often starts as a mild pain or pressure in the chest and is sometimes mistaken for indigestion. As it worsens, the pain is similar to angina, but more severe, and longer lasting. It may be accompanied by sweating, palpitations, breathlessness, vomiting or collapse. The pain may be felt in the central chest area and may radiate round to the back, up to the neck and jaw, or down the left arm.

Damage to the heart may lead to heart failure (a reduction in the heart's pumping efficiency). In severe cases, the victim's heart and breathing may stop. In this case cardiopulmonary resuscitation (CPR) can be attempted. This first-aid technique is a combination of mouth-to-mouth resuscitation and chest compressions and aims to keep oxygenated blood circulating in the body until an ambulance arrives. It is best carried out by those trained in the technique.

**Treatment** An aspirin given immediately to a conscious heart attack victim can improve blood flow and ease the symptoms. Medical staff may use drugs and/or defibrillation (electric shocks applied to the chest) to stabilise an erratic heart rhythm. This is followed by oxygen and strong painkillers such as morphine. In some cases, drugs to dissolve blood clots, and surgery to repair damaged heart muscle and improve blood flow through the heart, may be necessary. On recovery the heart attack victim must follow a rehabilitation programme incorporating diet, exercise and general health principles (see advice on 'preventing angina').

▶ *see also movement, massage, energy, natural, mind, relaxation therapies*

## Pulled muscle

Pain from a pulled chest muscle usually follows injury caused by a sudden strain, for example when lifting a heavy weight. The pain is felt along the line of the muscle as a dull ache or cramp-like pain. The muscle affected is often tender.

**Treatment** The application of cold compresses to the damaged muscle is a simple but effective treatment. An icepack, wrapped in a towel (see page 155), can be used in cases of severe inflammation. Manipulative treatments such as physiotherapy (see page 73) and rolfing (see page 72) can also be effective. Homeopaths recommend arnica for sprains and muscle aches: to make a tincture, mix 10 ml of arnica to 1 cup of water and apply it to the affected area. A poultice of ginger is also effective. Over-the-counter painkillers, such as aspirin, and liniment ointments and sprays are available from chemists.

▶ *see also manipulative, massage therapies*

## Shingles

Shingles occurs in people who have been previously exposed to the virus that causes chicken pox. The virus lies dormant in the nerve root and becomes active again when the body's immunity is low. People over the age of 50 are mainly affected by the disease because the efficiency of the immune system generally declines with age. Stress also affects the immune system and many people suffer from the disease after experiencing a period of emotional turmoil or pressure.

Shingles usually starts as a sharp burning pain that follows the route of the nerves around the chest, parallel to the ribs. The disorder causes a painful rash of small blisters on the skin. The pain of an attack can persist long after the blisters have healed. This chronic pain condition is called postherpetic neuralgia and is caused by damaged nerves producing strong pain impulses.

**Treatment** Conventional treatment for shingles includes antiviral drugs and painkillers. The early use of antiviral drugs can help minimise nerve damage, but if treatment is delayed postherpetic pain may be a major problem. Dabbing the sores gently with 2 drops of essential oil of lemon and geranium mixed with 1 cup of water can relieve the pain. Eating a well-balanced diet and increasing your intake of vitamins B, C, and E to boost your immune system can help to prevent the symptoms from recurring. The treatment of postherpetic neuralgia may involve specialised treatment from a pain clinic or acupuncturist.

▶ *see also massage, natural, relaxation therapies*

## Broken rib

A broken rib is usually caused by injury, for example, by a fall or a blow. In rare cases, however, it may result from excess stress on the rib cage brought on by coughing or even laughing. Pain is felt as a sharp, stabbing pain over the affected area. It is particularly severe if taking a deep breath or coughing.

**Treatment** The pain of a broken rib is usually treated with over-the-counter drugs such as ibuprofen, aspirin, paracetamol, or if necessary stronger drugs prescribed by a doctor. The rib must not be strapped, as this increases the risk of a chest infection developing. After the broken rib has healed sufficiently, treatment from a chiropractor or osteopath (see page 70) can help to rebuild muscle and ligament mobility.

▶ *see also manipulative, massage therapies*

---

### SELF HELP AND SHINGLES

There are a number of complementary treatments you can safely try at home to relieve the pain of shingles.

▶ *Mix equal parts of oat straw, St John's wort and skullcap tinctures and take 1 teaspoon four times a day.*

▶ *Mix carrot and celery juice with 1 tablespoon of parsley juice and drink.*

▶ *Soaking for half an hour to an hour in a bath heated to body temperature may help to calm the nervous system.*

▶ *TENS (transcutaneous electrical nerve stimulation, see page 83) is particularly effective for chronic nerve pain.*

▶ *Reflexology directed at the diaphragm, glands and the spine can be beneficial.*

---

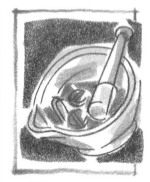

### ASPIRIN PASTE

An aspirin paste is a gentle way to relieve pain caused by shingles:

■ *Crush two aspirin tablets into a powder in a bowl.*

■ *Mix the crushed tablets with a plain skin cream until the tablets are dissolved.*

■ *Apply to the affected area.*

# ABDOMINAL PAIN

*The abdominal area is very sensitive to stress, and many recurrent abdominal pains respond well to relaxation therapies. Some kinds of pain, however, may indicate a serious problem.*

Abdominal pain may arise from the wall of the abdomen (skin, muscles and abdominal lining), the contents of the abdomen, or the nervous system. On occasion, abdominal pain may be referred from the organs of the chest or pelvis.

In many cases abdominal pain is short-term and can be safely treated at home. However, if the pain occurs together with other symptoms, such as vomiting or fever, you should consult a doctor immediately as these symptoms may indicate a serious condition such as appendicitis, stomach ulcer, or kidney infection. A precise description of the type and site of your pain will help your doctor to diagnose the underlying cause and suggest appropriate treatment. In general terms, there are five types of pain associated with the abdomen: generalised abdominal pain, pain of the upper middle abdomen, pain of the centre abdomen, pain of the lower abdomen, and pain of the rectal area.

## GENERALISED ABDOMINAL PAIN

Generalised abdominal pain is a term used to describe acute pain which affects the whole area of the abdomen. A serious cause of this wide-ranging pain is peritonitis (inflammation of the membrane called the peritoneum that lines the abdomen). The pain is acute and severe and requires urgent medical attention. Peritonitis is usually caused by infection which can occur when there is a leakage from the bowel due to perforation of an ulcer, a burst appendix, or rupture of an infected gall bladder. One of the most tell-tale signs of peritonitis is a board-like rigidity of the abdominal wall.

## PAINS IN THE UPPER MIDDLE ABDOMEN

Pains in the upper middle abdomen are mainly the result of problems in the lower oesophagus, stomach, liver, gall bladder, duodenum, pancreas, heart or lungs.

### Indigestion

The term 'indigestion' covers a variety of symptoms that may occur after eating a meal, from burping and a feeling of fullness to more painful symptoms. Pain is felt as a mild to moderate aching or burning sensation in the upper middle abdomen, which occasionally radiates to the back. While overeating is the most common cause of indigestion, stress, smoking and heavy drinking may all aggravate the condition.

## INSIDE THE ABDOMEN

The abdominal cavity is located between the lower ribs and the pubic area. It is lined by a membrane called the peritoneum and contains the digestive organs, the bladder and the rectum.

***ABDOMINAL PAIN***
*Pain in the abdomen often starts as a vague pain affecting the general abdominal area but then gradually can be pinpointed to a particular organ.*

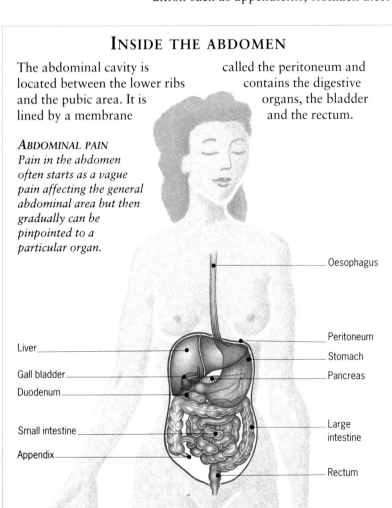

- Oesophagus
- Peritoneum
- Stomach
- Pancreas
- Large intestine
- Rectum
- Liver
- Gall bladder
- Duodenum
- Small intestine
- Appendix

**Treatment** Over-the-counter antacid drugs can usually relieve symptoms quickly, but they should not be used in the long-term as they may hide symptoms of serious disease. Aspirin should be avoided because it can irritate the stomach and in some cases cause gastric bleeding. Drinking milk and herbal teas such as peppermint, fennel or camomile after eating can help to ease discomfort. If you suffer frequently from indigestion and also observe other symptoms, such as vomiting, weight loss or a change in bowel movements, you should consult a doctor.

▶ *see also movement, massage, natural therapies*

## Peptic ulcer

A peptic ulcer is a break in the lining of the duodenum, stomach or oesophagus. It is caused by excess acid or a reduction in the mucus layer protecting the lining of the digestive tract, as a result of which the cells in the lining become eroded and an ulcer forms. The pain symptoms of a peptic ulcer are similar to indigestion but often more severe. The pain is commonly described as gnawing or burning.

Usually ulcers are caused by a bacterial infection. Chemicals secreted from the bacteria damage the lining of the intestine resulting in the formation of ulcers (see below). In these cases specialist treatment, including the use of antibiotics, is necessary.

**Treatment** If you have a peptic ulcer, you should be under the care of a medical specialist. Conventional medical treatment for

## HERBS AND INDIGESTION

There are a number of herbal treatments that can greatly relieve the symptoms of indigestion. For example, taking 25 to 50 g (1 to 2 oz) of aloe vera juice in a glass of water three times a day will soothe the digestive tract, while peppermint, taken as an infusion, can stabilise recurring indigestion problems. Or you could try a meadowsweet infusion to relieve nausea, reduce acidity and soothe the stomach's mucous membranes. Pour 1 cup of boiling water over 2 teaspoons of dried meadowsweet and leave to infuse for 15 minutes. Take the mixture three times a day.

ulcers is antacids, which work by neutralising stomach acids. Herbalists may recommend slippery elm bark powder taken as a broth one hour before meals and at bedtime. Homeopathic medicines may also be effective. If abdominal pain continues for several days or becomes more severe then medical advice is necessary.

There are also a wide number of self-help measures you can take to relieve the pain, the most important of which is to stop smoking. Alcohol, caffeine, aspirin and non-steroidal anti-inflammatory drugs all irritate the lining of the stomach and should be avoided. Eating two or three large meals a day may aggravate the condition and you may find that eating several small meals at regular intervals is beneficial. Finally stress, although unlikely to be the direct cause of an ulcer, can aggravate existing ulcers, so relaxation and meditation therapies should be considered.

## HOW A PEPTIC ULCER FORMS

Peptic ulcers are caused when acid from the stomach wall erodes the lining of the duodenum, oesophagus or stomach.

They can cause a burning aching pain in the abdomen and are usually accompanied by nausea and vomiting.

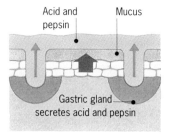

**The mucus** produced by the stomach lining normally protects the stomach from acid and pepsin secreted by the gastric glands

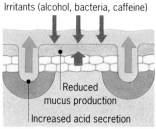

**Peptic ulcers** develop when there is reduced mucus production, increased acid secretion, or the stomach lining has been irritated

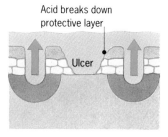

**The protective mucus layer** and mucus-secreting cells become eroded and an ulcer forms

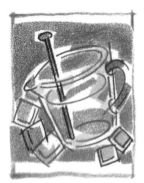

**DIARRHOEA: A SIMPLE SOLUTION**

Holiday diarrhoea attacks can be triggered by a change of diet or by consuming contaminated food or water. To ensure the disorder does not lead to severe dehydration, which is a potentially serious medical problem, take with you some sachets of rehydration salts (available from chemists). Alternatively you can make your own rehydration mixture as follows:

■ *Dissolve 1 teaspoon of salt and 8 teaspoons of sugar in 1 litre (1¼ pints) of boiled water and sip 3 litres of this mixture every day while symptoms last. You should keep to these proportions to ensure the remedy works effectively.*

Maintaining these self-help measures after your ulcer has cleared up should help to prevent a recurrence.

▶ *see also herbal, massage, movement therapies*

### Pancreatitis

Pancreatitis is inflammation of the pancreas and may be acute or chronic. The disorder is characterised by severe pain in the upper middle abdomen which in many cases radiates through to the middle of the back. Because the pancreas is an organ involved in food digestion, other symptoms may include problems with breaking down food, diarrhoea and weight loss.

Acute pancreatitis is often associated with excessive alcohol intake, but may also be caused by gallstones, trauma, metabolic disease or certain drugs. Chronic pancreatitis may cause diabetes: because the pancreas produces insulin, lack of which causes diabetes, any damage to the pancreas can cause a drop in insulin production.

**Treatment** Both acute and chronic pancreatitis require hospital inpatient treatment. In some cases removal of the pancreas may be necessary. This can lead to problems in digesting food, but these can be corrected by taking oral supplements of the digestive enzymes produced by the pancreas.

### Gall bladder disease

The gall bladder stores the bile necessary for digesting fats. Most painful disorders of the gall bladder are associated with gallstones which form when there is a chemical imbalance in the bile and some of its components solidify. If you experience acute pain in the upper part of the abdomen on the right side it may be due to inflammation of the gall bladder, known as cholecystitis. This happens when gallstones become trapped at the outlet of the gall bladder into the bile duct and the flow of bile is stopped. Other symptoms of cholecystitis are nausea, indigestion and jaundice, where the skin and whites of the eyes acquire a yellowish tint. If you experience gall bladder pain you should consult a doctor as soon as possible.

**Treatment** Some small gallstones may remain in the gall bladder for years without causing any problems. Others may pass harmlessly out of the body in the faeces. You can help to stimulate the flow of bile by incorporating bitter salads such as chicory and globe artichoke in your meals at least three times a week. Herbalists often recommend a daily cup of centaury tea to soothe inflammation. In addition, reducing your intake of animal fats and dairy products and taking no more than 2 units of alcohol a day can help to prevent gall bladder pain if you already suffer from it.

Stones that cause pain or inflammation of the gall bladder must be removed. If the stones are small enough they can be dissolved by drugs. Larger stones can be removed by endoscopy; this involves inserting a flexible viewing tube into the stomach and duodenum. Sometimes removal of the

## GALL BLADDER

The gall bladder is a small muscular sac that is located under the liver. Bile containing waste products from the liver is stored in the gall bladder until it enters the duodenum after a meal. If gallstones become trapped at the outlet of the gall bladder to the bile duct, they can cause extreme pain, blocking the flow of bile to the duodenum. To reduce the likelihood of developing gallstones, avoid becoming overweight and limit your intake of sugar and fat.

*GALL BLADDER PAIN*
*Gall bladder pain often radiates to the shoulder blades and is aggravated by deep breaths and pressure on the right abdomen.*

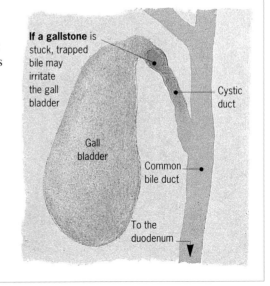

If a gallstone is stuck, trapped bile may irritate the gall bladder

Cystic duct

Gall bladder

Common bile duct

To the duodenum

gall bladder is recommended. This presents few problems as the digestive system can function normally without a gall bladder, although dietary changes to reduce the intake of fats may be recommended.

▶ *see also movement, massage, natural therapies*

### PAIN IN THE CENTRE ABDOMEN

Pain in the centre abdomen usually indicates an illness that is causing inflammation of the stomach or small intestine.

## Gastroenteritis

The commonest cause of pain in the centre abdomen is gastroenteritis, or inflammation of the stomach and intestines. It is commonly caused by consuming food or water that has been contaminated with food poisoning microorganisms. The pain is acute but often vague and the sufferer may also have a distended abdomen, nausea, and vomiting or diarrhoea. Usually the symptoms last only for a few days, but in more severe cases dehydration, shock and even collapse may occur. If severe pain persists for more than a few days in conjunction with vomiting, you should consult a doctor as the symptoms may indicate a more serious disease such as cholera or typhoid, which are mainly confined to developing countries.

**Treatment** It is vital to drink plenty of water in small amounts taken frequently to replace fluids lost through diarrhoea and vomiting and prevent dehydration. A rehydration mixture (see left) may be given, or flat lemonade can also be effective. Antibiotics may be necessary in some cases. After the diarrhoea and vomiting have subsided, eat plain wholefoods such as bananas and toast which can help to relieve gastric pains. Eating live yoghurt may also be beneficial as it replaces essential bacteria in the intestines.

### PAIN IN THE LOWER ABDOMEN

Pain in the lower abdomen usually indicates a problem of the large intestine (colon) such as inflammation (colitis), which is a feature of Crohn's disease (see below). Another cause of pain in this area is appendicitis, acute inflammation of the appendix. The appendix is a small closed tube branching off the colon. Disorders affecting the kidneys, the bladder, and the sex organs may also cause pain in the lower abdomen. These pains are covered in Chapter 7.

## Diverticulitis

If there are areas of weakness in the wall of the large intestine, the lining may be forced through the wall forming small sacs known as diverticula. Usually these sacs do not cause any problems. Sometimes, however, they can become inflamed resulting in a condition called diverticulitis. Abscesses may form in the tissues and bleeding may occur. The pain is often cramping, causing the affected part of the abdomen to feel rigid. Nausea, vomiting and a change in bowel habits (for instance diarrhoea or constipation) are frequently associated with the condition. In rare cases rupture of the sac may cause peritonitis (see page 108).

**Treatment** Diverticulitis is usually successfully treated with antibiotics. In more severe cases the affected part of the lower intestine may be removed by surgery. Slippery elm can help to soothe the pain of inflamed diverticula: mix 1 teaspoon of slippery elm powder with a little honey, then slowly add warm water while stirring to a consistency suitable for drinking or eating with a spoon. Take three times daily. Massaging the abdomen in the morning may also be helpful. You can help to prevent diverticulitis by including more fibre in your diet (but avoid foods with pips and seeds as these may collect in the sacs) and by drinking at least 2 litres (3½ pints) of water a day. This prevents constipation which can further inflame the intestine.

▶ *see also movement, massage, natural therapies*

---

### APPENDICITIS OR INDIGESTION?

Knowing how to spot the warning signs of appendicitis can be vital to ensure prompt medical treatment. If an inflamed appendix is not removed it may rupture, causing peritonitis (see page 108). In general, the initial pain of appendicitis is felt around the navel. When the abdominal lining becomes inflamed, the pain is focused on the right, just above the groin, and is severe, continuous and made worse by movement and coughing. Most sufferers lose their appetite, feel nauseous and may vomit or have diarrhoea. A mild inflammation known as a grumbling appendix may cause discomfort but is not a cause for concern.

---

## AIDING DIGESTION WITH MASSAGE

Massaging the abdomen can help to relax the abdominal muscles and aid digestion. You can do this in a chair while remaining fully clothed, but for best results try massaging directly onto the skin with essential oils mixed with a carrier oil. A drop of oil of peppermint or ginger in a teaspoon of almond oil is particularly effective.

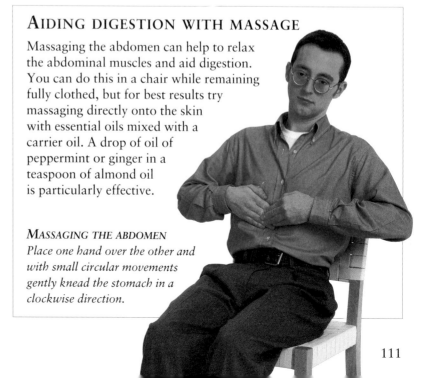

*MASSAGING THE ABDOMEN*
*Place one hand over the other and with small circular movements gently knead the stomach in a clockwise direction.*

## Crohn's disease

Crohn's disease is a chronic inflammatory condition of the large or small intestine. The condition causes severe spasms or continuous aching discomfort. It can also cause a lot of pain in the anus and rectum. The causes of the disease are not fully understood. Some authorities believe a diet high in processed foods may be a factor, while other theories suggest that the disease is an autoimmune response, in which the immune system attacks body tissues. This has been linked to infection and stress.

**Treatment** Hospital outpatient treatment is required for Crohn's disease. It can cause a deficiency in certain vitamins, so increasing your intake of vitamins A, B, D and beta-carotene may help to relieve some of the symptoms. Because stress can aggravate the condition, regular relaxation techniques and aromatherapy can be helpful. Hot and cold fomentations applied to the abdomen can improve the function of the intestine and relieve colic.

▶ *see also movement, massage, energy, natural, mind, relaxation therapies*

## Irritable bowel syndrome

Irritable bowel syndrome is a painful condition of the lower intestine causing irregular bouts of diarrhoea or constipation or alternating bouts of both. Sufferers develop cramp-like abdominal pains and may have a feeling of distension in the abdomen. As in Crohn's disease, the symptoms are aggravated by emotional stress. Little is known about the causes of the condition although it is thought that abnormal functioning of the muscles in the large intestine may contribute. Food intolerance, specifically an intolerance to lactose (a sugar found in milk), may be a factor in the development of the illness.

**Treatment** Although irritable bowel syndrome has no cure, you can take steps to alleviate the painful symptoms with a variety of treatments. Eating a well-balanced diet with a high intake of fibre-rich foods (a daily intake of 18 g of fibre is recommended) can help to prevent attacks. Good sources include fresh apples, pears and dates. Although bran was formerly recommended for the condition, some sufferers

## YOGA FOR REGULAR BOWEL MOVEMENTS

To establish regular bowel movements it can be helpful to start each day with this simple yoga exercise. If you are reasonably supple, you could extend the two-step exercise below into the 'half shoulder stand' (right). If you have a back disorder or suffer some other serious condition, consult your doctor before attempting these exercises.

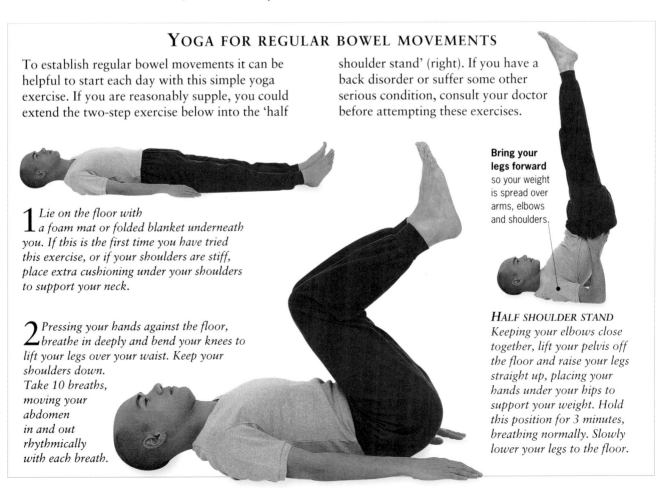

1 *Lie on the floor with a foam mat or folded blanket underneath you. If this is the first time you have tried this exercise, or if your shoulders are stiff, place extra cushioning under your shoulders to support your neck.*

2 *Pressing your hands against the floor, breathe in deeply and bend your knees to lift your legs over your waist. Keep your shoulders down. Take 10 breaths, moving your abdomen in and out rhythmically with each breath.*

**Bring your legs forward** so your weight is spread over arms, elbows and shoulders.

*HALF SHOULDER STAND*
*Keeping your elbows close together, lift your pelvis off the floor and raise your legs straight up, placing your hands under your hips to support your weight. Hold this position for 3 minutes, breathing normally. Slowly lower your legs to the floor.*

have found that bran actually aggravates their condition and it is generally best avoided. Eating live natural yoghurt will help to keep the balance of bacteria in the gut healthy, which should also help the condition. It may be better to avoid coffee and chocolate because they contain a chemical that causes contraction of the bowel and can lead to abdominal pain. At least 2 litres (3½ pints) of fluid should be drunk every day. Herbalists suggest drinking peppermint tea rather than tea or coffee after eating, as it has a soothing effect on the stomach and intestines. Aromatherapy massage (see page 79) can be effective as it reduces stress and helps to soothe muscle spasms.

▶ *see also movement, massage, energy, natural, mind, relaxation therapies*

## Constipation and flatulence

A sedentary lifestyle and poor dietary habits can lead to irregular bowel movements. When the faeces are hard, it becomes more difficult to excrete them from the bowel, resulting in constipation, flatulence and considerable lower abdominal discomfort. If you experience a sudden change in your normal pattern of bowel movements which you cannot account for, it may indicate a condition requiring further investigation.

**Treatment**  Eating plenty of fibre such as bran, wholemeal bread, brown rice and fresh fruit, and drinking plenty of water (at least seven glasses a day), is vital for keeping faeces soft. Regular exercise such as walking, cycling or swimming, and yoga exercises every morning (see left) help to stimulate bowel movement. The discomfort of constipation can be relieved by taking 2 teaspoons of psyllium or ground linseed in your cereal or coffee. If the constipation attack is an isolated one, dried prunes, figs or apricots are excellent natural laxatives.

Although some amount of flatulence is normal, it can become a problem if large amounts of undigested food pass into the intestine. The bacteria that settle on this food produce excess gas. Some foods, such as bran, beans, broccoli, cauliflower, Brussels sprouts, cabbage, dark beer and fizzy drinks are more 'gassy' than others. If you suffer from chronic flatulence it may help to try eliminating some of these foods to try to pinpoint the cause. As beans and peas are also a rich source of fibre and protein, it's best not to leave them out of your

diet completely. One way of making them less gaseous is to cook them according to the following method. Place the beans in a bowl of water and soak overnight. Drain the soaked beans, cover with fresh water and cook for 30 minutes. Drain and replace the water again and cook for another 30 minutes. Finally, drain once more, replace with fresh water and cook until tender.

▶ *see also movement, massage, natural therapies*

## Stitch

The term 'stitch' is used to describe the pain that is felt in the side during exercise, often following a heavy meal. The condition is caused by insufficient blood supply to the muscles because blood has been diverted to the intestines to aid digestion, or because the exercise is too intense. If the pain of a stitch persists the muscle may have developed a spasm or possibly a tear.

**Treatment**  If you have a stitch during exercise, stop exercising and gently stretch the affected area. Breathe deeply for a few minutes and the pain should subside. You can help to prevent a stitch by avoiding eating heavy meals prior to exercise. Always allow at least one hour to digest your food before engaging in physical activity. Eating meals high in complex carbohydrates, such as pasta, at least an hour before you exercise may also help to prevent the onset of stitch. Don't exercise for too long at any one time, and make sure that the exercises are within your fitness level.

▶ *see also movement, massage, natural therapies*

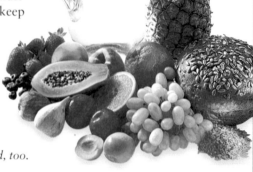

## FOODS TO FIGHT CONSTIPATION

Although bowel movements vary according to the individual, you should make sure that your diet contains sufficient dietary fibre and that you are drinking plenty of liquids. Both are necessary to keep the faeces soft so they can pass painlessly through the colon.

***FIBRE AND FLUIDS***
*Fibre eases constipation and is found in fruits, vegetables, grains and beans. Drink lots of fluid, too.*

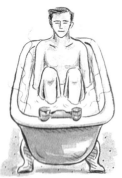

***IMPROVISING A SITZBATH***
*You can enjoy sitzbath therapy in your bath at home. First fill the bath with about 10 cm (4 in) of warm water. Sit in the bath, keep your knees up and splash water onto the abdomen. Stay in for 15 minutes, then refill the bath with cold water and rinse. You can also add herbs or oils to the hot bath (see below).*

## RECTAL PAINS

The rectum is the lowest part of the large intestine and connects the intestine to the anus. A variety of painful disorders such as inflammation, polyps (growths) and cancer may affect the rectum and anal canal.

### Haemorrhoids

Haemorrhoids, commonly known as piles, are swollen blood vessels in the lining of the anus. They may occur inside the anus or close to the anal opening. They can lead to intense itching and pain and sometimes bleed when faeces are passed. They are caused by increased pressure on the blood vessels in the anus, for example, when straining to pass hard faeces, or when lifting heavy items, or during pregnancy.

**Treatment** Applying witch hazel to the sensitive area may give some relief from the pain of piles or you can make your own ointment to relieve the pain: simmer 30 g (1 oz) of pilewort with 200 g (6½ oz) of vaseline for 10 minutes. Naturopaths may recommend a sitzbath to relieve the pain caused by problems such as piles or tears in the anus caused by straining to pass hard faeces. A sitzbath has two sections, one containing hot water and another containing cold water. The patient sits in the hot water with feet in the cold water for two or three minutes and then the procedure is reversed for one minute. You can also improvise your own sitzbath (see left). In some cases, an injection is given to make haemorrhoids shrink. Surgery is only necessary if haemorrhoids are very large or troublesome.

Constipation is one of the main causes of piles – altering your diet to produce softer faeces can alleviate the pain considerably (see page 113). Also, try to avoid foods that cause irritation such as coffee and spices. Consuming sufficient liquids to soften the faeces is important – aim to drink at least seven glasses of water a day. Natural laxatives such as prunes, figs and raisins may help prevent the pain caused by straining.

▶ *see also massage, natural, relaxation therapies*

---

## SOOTHING HAEMORRHOIDS WITH HERBS

Camomile has long been recognised for its ability to soothe sore, inflamed or itchy skin. Adding it to a bath will help heal skin damaged by haemorrhoids.

Haemorrhoids can also be soothed by adding to a bath 4 drops of essential oils of both peppermint and cypress, with 2 tablespoons of bicarbonate of soda.

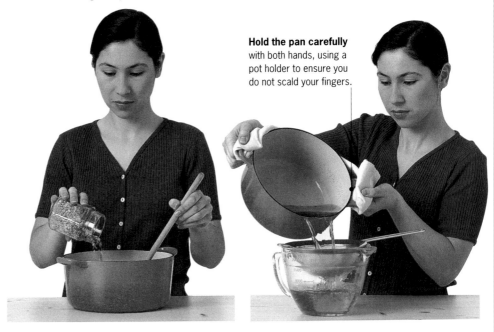

**Hold the pan carefully** with both hands, using a pot holder to ensure you do not scald your fingers.

**1** *Mix 20g (¾oz) of camomile flowers with 3 litres (5 pints) cold water in a large pan. Bring to boil. Cover and simmer for 10 mins.*

**2** *Strain the liquid carefully into a bowl. Add the liquid to the warm bath water, mix well and climb in.*

# CHAPTER 7

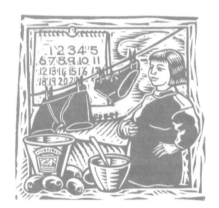

# MALE AND FEMALE COMPLAINTS

*Disorders relating to the female and male reproductive and urinary systems can threaten fertility and health as well as causing severe pain. In most cases the first course of action must be to seek medical opinion, but there are natural remedies, both old and new, which you can use together with your doctor's advice not only to ease pain but also to prevent conditions from recurring.*

# WOMEN'S COMPLAINTS

*By taking good care of your body and using natural therapies, you can often avoid or relieve many painful disorders affecting the breasts and the reproductive and urinary systems.*

Many of the more serious disorders affecting women – such as breast and cervical cancer, and infections such as chlamydia, a common cause of female infertility – can be treated successfully and leave no lasting damage if caught in the early stages. Learning about possible causes of female disorders will help you to take steps to avoid such problems in the future. Similarly, being able to recognise the warning signs of illness means that you can seek early treatment and so improve the chances of a complete cure.

## PAIN AND THE FEMALE BODY

The first step in the early detection of disorders is to get to know your body: how it normally looks, feels and reacts. Examine your body regularly for any abnormal changes such as menstrual irregularities, the sudden appearance of lumps, swellings or skin blemishes, or any other warning signals your body may reveal.

▶ *Headaches may be frequent prior to menstruation due to hormonal changes.*

▶ *The breasts are susceptible to swelling and tenderness before menstruation.*

▶ *The lower abdomen contains the female reproductive organs which may be affected by growths, infection, abnormal bleeding and inflammation.*

▶ *The vaginal area is prone to infection and inflammation.*

*A HEALTHY BODY*
*Regular exercise can do much to prevent and relieve many painful disorders.*

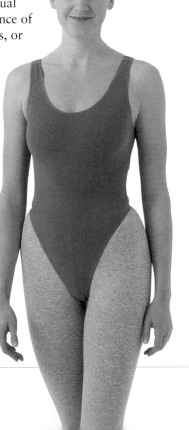

### BREAST PAIN
Most women suffer from breast pain at some time in their lives. The most common are premenstrual breast pain, a chronic condition, and mastitis, an acute disorder.

### Premenstrual breast pain
Before menstruation the breasts may feel tender and 'lumpy' and in some women the pain may be severe. The condition is linked to hormonal changes in the body prior to menstruation: raised levels of oestrogen in the blood causes water retention in the breasts, making them feel full and tender. This kind of pain usually disappears once menstruation begins, but if it continues, consult a doctor.

**Treatment** Premenstrual pain can often be treated by simple painkillers. Massaging the breasts with geranium oil or adding a few drops to a bath can be soothing. Evening primrose oil taken in capsule form may be effective at reducing pain. To help to counteract water retention you can try natural diuretics such as freshly chopped parsley. In some cases, hormone therapy may be required to alleviate the condition.
▶ *See also massage, energy, natural therapies*

### Mastitis
Mastitis, or inflammation of the breast tissue, is usually associated with breast-feeding and is most often caused by bacterial infection entering via small cracks in the nipples. The breast becomes red, painful and swollen. In some cases, an abscess may form in the breast leading to fever.

**Treatment** The affected breast should be fully emptied, either by breastfeeding or expressing the milk. Antibiotic pills are prescribed, but if an abscess forms surgery is required to drain it. Vitamin E cream can help to soothe and treat cracked nipples.
▶ *See also massage, energy, natural therapies*

## ABDOMINAL PAIN

Any persistent new pain, especially if it is accompanied by other symptoms, such as bleeding between periods, increased menstrual bleeding, pain during sexual intercourse or abnormal vaginal discharge, could be an indication of a more serious condition and you should seek a doctor's opinion as soon as possible. Alternatively, you might prefer to visit a gynaecologist or a well woman clinic. For information on abdominal pains, other than those caused by gynaecological problems, see page 108.

## Premenstrual syndrome (PMS)

The physical and psychological changes experienced by women in the days before menstruation are known as premenstrual syndrome (PMS). The physical symptoms include breast tenderness, swelling of the abdomen, abdominal pains, headaches, appetite changes and cramps. Psychological symptoms include depression, tearfulness, anxiety, irritability and lack of sexual interest. Symptoms may start up to 14 days prior to a period and disappear at the onset of menstrual bleeding. Distressing and sometimes severe enough to produce disruption to work and family life, PMS is complex and there is still no agreement over its definition and treatment.

**Treatment** Evening primrose oil capsules may be of benefit. Herbalists recommend preparations of agnus castus and diuretic herbs. Naturopaths may suggest vitamin $B_6$ and magnesium supplements to calm the nerves. Daily infusions of camomile may reduce water retention. Exercise such as swimming and yoga may also be of value.
▶ *See also massage, movement, energy therapies*

## Painful periods

Dysmenorrhoea, or painful periods, is most often caused by changes in hormone levels, and in particular to an abnormal increase in prostaglandins. Pain is generally worse during the first two days of menstruation and sufferers usually experience cramp-like pains in the abdomen, back pain and muscle spasms of the uterus. However, painful periods may also indicate a gynaecological disorder such as pelvic inflammatory disease or endometriosis (see page 118). The intra-uterine contraceptive device (IUD or coil) may also lead to painful periods.

**Treatment** Progestogen may be prescribed to correct the hormonal imbalance. The oestrogen-progestogen oral contraceptive pill is effective by causing lighter, shorter periods. Hot and cold fomentations (see page 87) or a hot-water bottle placed on the abdomen and lower back can help to relieve period pains. Massaging the abdomen with oils (see page 111) or taking a hot bath to which a few drops of lavender oil have been added can also be soothing.

Painkillers such as aspirin and ibuprofen that inhibit the release of prostaglandins may be effective. Magnesium supplements help to reduce cramping. Herbalists may

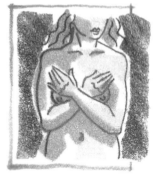

## LOOKING AFTER YOUR BREASTS

By maintaining a healthy lifestyle you can help to avoid breast disorders:

■ *Cut down on salt and salty foods to reduce water retention.*

■ *Eat foods rich in vitamin A to soothe pain and vitamin $B_6$ to reduce water retention.*

■ *Drink alcohol only in moderation, avoid cigarettes and decrease intake of fats to reduce the risk of cancer.*

■ *Invest in well-fitting support bras to prevent sore chest muscles.*

■ *Examine your breasts regularly for lumps and other abnormalities.*

## DIETARY CHANGES

Dietary changes around ten days before menstruation can help to alleviate some of the painful symptoms associated with PMS. For example, cutting back on the amount of sugar and salt in your diet may reduce breast pain, and decreasing your caffeine intake can help to reduce anxiety and irritability.

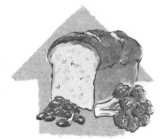
Increase your intake of fibre by eating wholemeal bread and green vegetables to avoid constipation

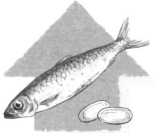
Eat regular meals rich in vitamins and minerals to maintain blood sugar levels and promote health

Reduce your intake of caffeine, which can make you feel tense, anxious, nervous and irritable

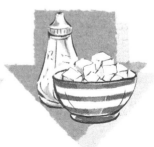
Cut down on salt and junk foods high in fat and sugar to reduce sluggishness and bloated feelings

## EXERCISES TO REDUCE MENSTRUAL PAIN

Cramp-like pain or discomfort prior to or during menstruation, a condition known as dysmenorrhoea, is common and may be severe enough to affect work or leisure. If you frequently suffer from menstrual cramps, exercise may help to relieve the pain.

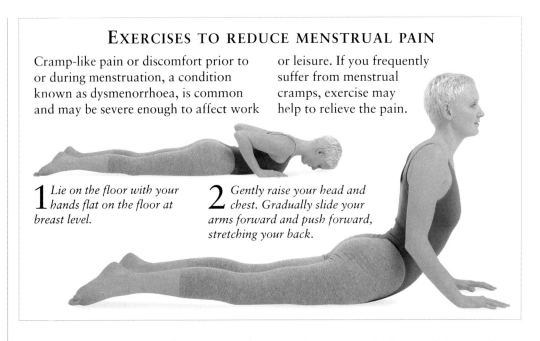

**1** *Lie on the floor with your hands flat on the floor at breast level.*

**2** *Gently raise your head and chest. Gradually slide your arms forward and push forward, stretching your back.*

also prescribe warming and antispasmodic herbs such as ginger and wild yam.

▶ *See also massage, movement, energy therapies*

### Pelvic inflammatory disease

Pelvic inflammatory disease (PID) is an infection of the female reproductive organs causing pain in the lower abdomen, fever, irregular periods and abnormal discharge. If untreated, PID may lead to chronic pain, heavy periods and infertility.

**Treatment** PID sufferers are usually treated with antibiotics. Severe cases may require hospital admission and sometimes surgery. Naturopaths recommend hydrotherapy to improve the circulation, plus vitamin supplements to strengthen the immune system.

▶ *See also massage, movement, energy therapies*

### Endometriosis

In this condition, pieces of endometrium (the lining of the uterus) become attached to organs outside the uterus, such as the Fallopian tubes. The tissue continues to react to hormonal changes, causing painful cysts and excessive menstrual bleeding. In some cases, it may lead to infertility.

**Treatment** Mild pain can be relieved by anti-inflammatory painkillers, such as ibuprofen. Drugs may be given to prevent menstruation, and surgery may be necessary to remove cysts. In severe cases, removal of the uterus and ovaries may be considered, particularly for older women. The condition may clear up with pregnancy.

▶ *See also massage, energy, natural therapies*

### Uterine fibroids

Uterine fibroids are benign tumours of the uterus that can occur without symptoms. Large fibroids can give rise to colicky pain, heavy periods, pelvic pain, painful intercourse and complications in pregnancy.

## THE FEMALE REPRODUCTIVE SYSTEM

The organs in the female pelvic cavity enable a woman to have sexual intercourse, produce eggs and develop a foetus, and to give birth. Painful disorders affecting this area may be caused by a variety of problems ranging from hormonal imbalances and structural abnormalities to infections and growths.

***WARNING SIGNS***
*Painful symptoms of the lower abdomen may indicate an infection or other disorder and should never be ignored.*

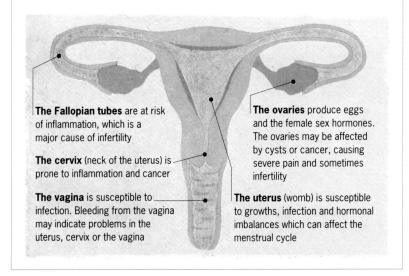

**The Fallopian tubes** are at risk of inflammation, which is a major cause of infertility

**The cervix** (neck of the uterus) is prone to inflammation and cancer

**The vagina** is susceptible to infection. Bleeding from the vagina may indicate problems in the uterus, cervix or the vagina

**The ovaries** produce eggs and the female sex hormones. The ovaries may be affected by cysts or cancer, causing severe pain and sometimes infertility

**The uterus** (womb) is susceptible to growths, infection and hormonal imbalances which can affect the menstrual cycle

## SEX THERAPIST

Sex therapy is a form of treatment, mainly involving counselling, that helps a couple to overcome sexual problems which are primarily psychological in origin. The therapy is based on the assumption that sexual problems arise from a range of causes, past and present, but the problems are maintained by the situation that the couple currently find themselves in. The therapist aims to modify the situation by clarifying the nature of the problems and exploring the factors contributing to the dysfunctional relationship. A couple will usually visit a sex therapist together, although individual consultations are possible. After the couple have been assessed it is hoped that they will have a better understanding of their problems and how to approach them. For example, the sex therapist might help a woman to identify emotional problems causing painful sex, or a man to discover the underlying cause of impotence or premature ejaculation. A simple explanation of sexual anatomy may help a couple to understand the physical causes of a sexual problem. The therapist can then discuss a programme of treatment.

**Treatment** In severe cases, surgery may be necessary. Fibroids may sometimes respond to homeopathic remedies.

▶ *See also massage, natural, relaxation therapies*

### Ovarian cysts

Ovarian cysts are fluid-filled sacs that form in an ovary. They may cause abdominal pain, especially if the cyst places pressure on the bladder, or ruptures or twists, and heavy and painful periods. Most are benign but around five per cent are malignant.

**Treatment** Surgery is often necessary to remove the cyst. Naturopaths believe cysts are part of the body's attempt to detoxify itself and suggest drinking 2 litres (3½ pints) of water a day, and also avoiding highly processed foods, alcohol and caffeine to help in this process.

▶ *See also massage, energy, relaxation therapies*

### Bartholinitis

Bartholin's glands are two glands at the opening of the vagina that help to lubricate the vulva during intercourse. These glands can become infected causing bartholinitis.

**Treatment** Antibiotic drugs are used to fight the infection and painkillers will ease the pain. If an abscess has formed, surgery may be necessary to drain it. In severe cases the gland may have to be removed. This does not affect the lubrication of the vagina as other glands also secrete lubricants.

▶ *See also massage, energy, natural therapies*

### PAIN DURING SEXUAL INTERCOURSE

Pain during sexual intercourse may affect the vagina or be felt deep in the pelvic area. It may be caused by a pelvic disorder, vaginal damage, or psychological problems.

### Vaginismus

Some women may experience involuntary contraction of the muscles around the vagina, making sex impossible or painful. This may be due to fear of penetration or follow vaginal damage caused in childbirth.

**Treatment** If the problem is psychological, sex therapy (see above) may be necessary. Relaxation methods such as yoga, aromatherapy and massage can help. Damage due to childbirth should start to heal within ten days but may stay painful for several weeks.

▶ *See also massage, movement, mind therapies*

### Vaginal atrophy

Vaginal atrophy, or thinning of the vaginal tissue following menopause, causes vaginal dryness and may lead to painful intercourse.

**Treatment** Hormone cream may help, as well as using vaginal lubricants such as K-Y jelly, vegetable oils or vitamin E cream.

▶ *See also natural, mind, relaxation therapies*

### INFLAMED BARTHOLIN'S GLANDS

Ducts leading to the glands can become blocked, causing pain and swelling. In some cases, a painful abscess may form. Other glands in the vagina can also get infected, a condition known as vestibulitis, making intercourse painful and sometimes impossible.

*PAIN RELIEF*
*Some women suffer repeated bouts of inflamed Bartholin's glands. A warm bath followed by aloe vera gel applied to the inflamed area often provides relief.*

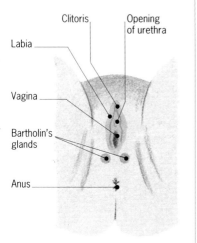

Clitoris
Opening of urethra
Labia
Vagina
Bartholin's glands
Anus

# PAIN RELIEF AND CHILDBIRTH

Pain management during childbirth is a very personal issue. The use of painkilling drugs is widespread and for many women is essential for pain control. Becoming informed about the drugs available is essential so that you can make the right choices during the birth. However, many women prefer the concept of a natural birth with minimal medical intervention and the avoidance of drugs. The use of relaxation techniques and being well informed about the birth process are both key features of natural pain control.

## NATURAL TECHNIQUES

Thorough preparation for childbirth helps to reduce the need for pain relief. Attending antenatal classes, exercising to strengthen your back and pelvic muscles, practising relaxation and breathing techniques, and seeking emotional support can all help to reduce the fear of labour so the pain is not experienced so acutely, and improve your ability to cope with it.

During contractions, many women find that walking around helps to distract the mind and that kneeling, squatting or sitting can all be more comfortable than lying down. Massaging the back and buttocks with

*EXERCISING THE PELVIC MUSCLES*
*Strengthening the pelvic muscles through exercise can help to improve your stamina during labour.*

**Lie flat** with arms at your sides and knees bent. While pressing your back against the floor, tighten and then relax the muscles used to control urine flow. Repeat ten times.

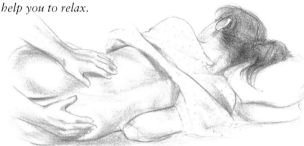

*COMFORTABLE LABOUR*
*Ask your partner to massage your back during labour to soothe the pain and help you to relax.*

talc can also be effective. Between contractions, the partner should use slow, firm strokes working from the centre of the back to the sides. During contractions, light circular strokes on the base of the spine are the most effective.

Massaging the acupressure point between the inner anklebone and the Achilles tendon may provide some pain relief. Use your thumb and massage the point for 60 seconds, first on one foot, then the other.

Acupuncture (see page 80) may also make labour easier and is becoming increasingly available. Another popular technique is transcutaneous nerve stimulation, or TENS (see page 83). This provides mild pain relief in early labour, but may be less effective in later stages.

## ORTHODOX TECHNIQUES

Oxygen and nitrous oxide ('laughing gas') is commonly used for pain relief in labour, and is effective for 50-60 per cent of women. It also has the advantage of being self-administered. Narcotic drugs such as pethidine provide some degree of pain relief for a few hours but are not effective for all women. Side effects include nausea, vomiting and drowsiness in the mother. The baby may have problems breathing after delivery, but this is remedied with medication.

An epidural is the most reliable form of orthodox pain relief during labour. Side effects are rare, although women may suffer headaches or backache afterwards. There is minimal effect on the baby. A woman may feel less in control of her labour, however, and forceps deliveries are more common as the mother doesn't feel the same urge to push.

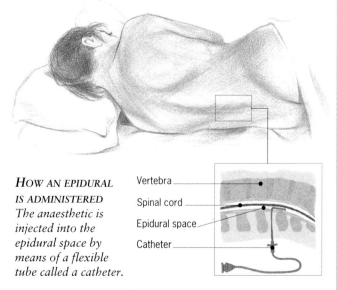

*HOW AN EPIDURAL IS ADMINISTERED*
*The anaesthetic is injected into the epidural space by means of a flexible tube called a catheter.*

Vertebra
Spinal cord
Epidural space
Catheter

# MEN'S COMPLAINTS

*Disorders of the male reproductive system – the testicles, penis and prostate – can cause pain and embarrassment. If left untreated, they may put a man's health and fertility at risk.*

Disorders affecting the male genitals often go untreated for too long because, through fear or embarrassment, many men are reluctant to discuss sexual health matters with their doctor. A knowledge of the causes and consequences of such disorders, and of the orthodox and complementary methods used in their treatment, can help men to prevent or alleviate many complaints which might otherwise cause psychological as well as physical pain.

### PENIS PROBLEMS

The male sex organ, the penis, can be the source of considerable pain if the nerves, blood vessels or skin become damaged through infection or, more rarely, injury.

### Paraphimosis

An overtight foreskin (phimosis) which does not retract easily can cause painful erections and discomfort during sexual intercourse. In paraphimosis the foreskin is so tight that it becomes caught behind the head of the penis, or glans, causing swelling and pain.
**Treatment**  The swelling may be reduced by applying an ice pack. The foreskin can then be returned to its normal position by squeezing the glans. In some cases, minor surgery may be needed to cut the foreskin.
▶ *See also massage, energy, natural therapies*

### Priapism

Very rarely, an erection may occur without sexual stimulation and not subside with time. Known as priapism, this painful condition is due to disease or damage to the blood vessels supplying the penis.
**Treatment**  If an erection fails to subside then medical treatment should be sought immediately to avoid permanent damage to the penis. Treatment usually involves taking blood from the penis to reduce the erection.
▶ *See also massage, energy, natural therapies*

### Balanitis

An uncircumcised penis may become infected under the foreskin, making the area red, moist and itchy. Known as balanitis, the condition may be caused by infection, irritation from clothes, or an allergic reaction of the skin to a chemical in soaps or condoms.
**Treatment**  Balanitis is usually treated with ointment or antibiotics. Applying aloe vera gel to the affected area after washing and drying the penis may also be effective.
▶ *See also massage, energy, natural therapies*

## PAIN AND THE MALE BODY

The male reproductive organs and urinary tract together form a complex system which can be prone to a variety of painful disorders. The older male, in particular, may suffer from pain associated with prostate disorders.

▶ *The bladder is susceptible to infection, which may cause pain on passing urine.*

▶ *The prostate gland lies below the bladder. As it gradually enlarges with age, it may start to press on the bladder, causing pain and obstructing the flow of urine.*

▶ *The penis carries urine and semen to the outside. It may be affected by infection or inflammation.*

▶ *The testicles are extremely sensitive – even the slightest injury can cause severe pain. They may also become swollen or inflamed.*

*STRESS AND HEALTH*
*Many men neglect their emotional health. Relaxation and stress reduction play an essential role in the relief of illnesses.*

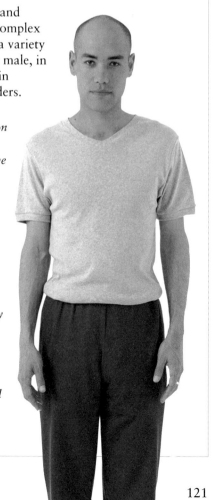

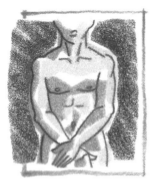

## LOOKING AFTER YOUR PENIS

Healthy diet, exercise and good hygiene practice can help to avoid some of the disorders that affect male sex organs:

■ *Always wash the penis carefully when having a bath or shower. If uncircumcised, pull back the foreskin to clean the head of the penis and avoid a build-up of oil secretions called smegma.*

■ *At least once a week, massage the penis with essential oil of tea tree – an antibacterial agent – mixed with a carrier such as almond oil.*

■ *Exercise regularly to improve sex drive and general performance.*

■ *Keep the genital muscles (which control urine flow) well toned by practising squeezing the muscles for 3 seconds and then releasing.*

## ANATOMY OF THE PENIS

The penis, the male sex organ, is susceptible to inflammation and infection through unprotected sexual intercourse and poor hygiene practices. Infection is most likely to develop underneath the foreskin in uncircumcised men, and in the urethra, the tube that conducts semen and urine along the penis. Using condoms and regular washing can help to prevent many of the disorders that may affect the penis.

*CROSS-SECTION OF THE PENIS*
*The penis is the male organ through which semen and urine pass out of the body. The penis consists of three groups of spongy tissue. When a man becomes sexually aroused these tissues fill with blood under pressure, expand and lengthen to produce an erection.*

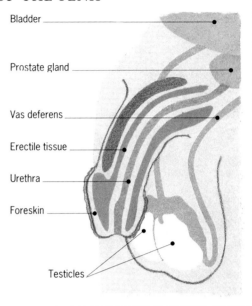

Bladder
Prostate gland
Vas deferens
Erectile tissue
Urethra
Foreskin
Testicles

## Peyronie's disease

With Peyronie's disease, part of the sheath of fibrous connective tissue in the penis becomes thicker, causing an abnormal bend during erection. In some cases the penis becomes so distorted that intercourse is painful or even impossible. Little is known about the causes of this disease, which usually affects men over the age of 40. Even if the condition persists, pain on erection usually eases within 12-18 months.

**Treatment** Corticosteroids are usually prescribed to alleviate the pain. If the condition persists, surgery may be necessary.
▶ *See also energy, natural therapies*

### TESTICLE PAIN

Hanging behind and below the penis in a pouch of skin called the scrotum, the testicles, or testes, produce sperm and the male sex hormone testosterone. They are vulnerable to injury and pain, especially during sporting activities. A heavy blow to the testicles may tear the testicle wall causing severe pain and bleeding into the scrotum, and will require surgery to repair.

There are a range of disorders that can affect the testicles (see below), not all of which cause pain. Cancer of the testicle, for example, is usually painless. You should see a doctor if you experience inflammation or abnormal pain in the testicles or notice any abnormal swelling when carrying out a regular testicular examination (see page 124).

## Hydrocele

Occasionally fluid can accumulate in the scrotum around the testicles due to inflammation, infection or injury, and may cause a painless swelling.

**Treatment** The fluid may be drained off under a local anaesthetic. If the problem persists, surgery may be necessary.
▶ *See also energy, natural therapies*

## Varicocele

Aching in the scrotum may be due to a varicocele, a usually painless condition almost exclusively affecting the left testicle. The condition is caused by a valve in the testicular vein failing to close properly, so that blood drains back and collects in the vein.

**Treatment** Any pain associated with varicocele can usually be relieved with simple painkillers such as paracetamol. Surgery may be necessary to tie off the swollen vein. Supporting the scrotum with tighter underpants or an athletic support can be helpful.
▶ *See also energy, natural therapies*

## Torsion of the testicle

The spermatic cord, which connects the testicle to the bladder, can suddenly twist, obstructing the blood supply. The pain is acute and often very severe.

**Treatment** You should consult a doctor immediately, as surgery may be necessary to restore the blood supply to the testes.
▶ *See also energy, natural therapies*

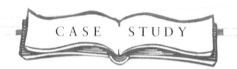

CASE STUDY

# Man with Painful Urination

*Once young people get caught up in the social whirl of student life, it is easy for them to fall into the trap of excess drinking and smoking, poor diet, casual sexual affairs and insufficient sleep. The body may react to this unhealthy lifestyle by becoming prone to infection and developing chronic painful disorders that can be difficult to treat and tend to recur.*

Alan is a single, outgoing 22-year-old student who enjoys socialising with friends most evenings and living on a diet of junk food. Recently he has experienced an aching pain in his groin, genitals and lower back and he constantly has the urge to pass urine. The pain has gradually become more severe and he has noticed his urine is now cloudy and contains some blood. His doctor prescribed antibiotics but Alan's pain continued, so he was referred to a urology specialist who diagnosed inflammation of the prostate (prostatitis). In spite of a further course of antibiotics the symptoms persisted. Because of the constant pain, Alan finds it difficult to concentrate and his social life and studying are suffering.

## WHAT SHOULD ALAN DO?

Alan should consult a pain specialist at a non-acute pain management centre. This gives access to a multidisciplinary health team offering treatments such as TENS, acupuncture and hypnotherapy. Alan should also look at his diet and general lifestyle, which may be adding to his problems. He is not in a steady relationship but has had several casual affairs, which may have put him at risk of a sexually transmitted infection. Psychologists at the centre can offer advice on cutting down on drinking, smoking and late nights. Alan should begin to exercise regularly, walking every day as much as his pain allows. A course of antidepressants may help to relieve the pain.

**DIET**
*Spicy foods, caffeine, alcohol, tobacco and foods high in fat and sugar can irritate the prostate and negate the effects of essential nutrients such as zinc and vitamins C and E.*

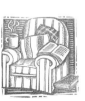

**LIFESTYLE**
*Lack of sleep and broken rest patterns, together with excessive smoking, drinking and irregular meal times, can have a detrimental effect on the immune system, leading to chronic or recurring infections.*

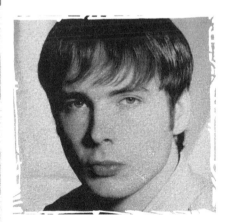

**SEX LIFE**
*Inflamed prostate is often caused by an infection such as chlamydia, which can be passed on during sexual intercourse.*

## Action Plan

**DIET**
*Avoid alcohol, which irritates the bladder. Increase water intake to eight glasses per day to dilute the urine and wash out bacteria.*

**LIFESTYLE**
*Make time for relaxation exercises to reduce stress levels, and restore balance to a hectic lifestyle by sticking to a regular schedule that ensures adequate sleep.*

**SEX LIFE**
*Follow safer sex practices, such as always using a condom if you have multiple sexual partners, or if your partner's sexual history is unknown to you.*

## HOW THINGS TURNED OUT FOR ALAN

The antidepressants made Alan feel drowsy and he found it harder to pass urine. TENS proved to be helpful but Alan did not feel that it provided a long-term solution. However, acupuncture and relaxation were effective and counselling has increased his self-esteem. He is now in a steady relationship, so, with an improved diet, regular exercise and a supportive girlfriend, his lifestyle has become more stable and his health has greatly improved.

## Testicular examination

An abnormal swelling of the testes may indicate a serious problem such as testicular cancer and should be reported to a doctor as soon as possible. You should regularly examine both testicles – cancers are usually firm to the touch and neither tender nor painful when pressed.

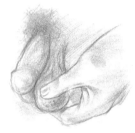

***EXAMINING THE TESTICLES***
*Hold the scrotum gently and feel the entire surface of the testicle for any abnormal lump.*

## Epididymitis

The epididymis, the coiled tube that carries sperm to the penis, can become infected causing a dull, aching pain and, in severe cases, inflammation of the scrotum. The pain may be worse during ejaculation and the semen may contain blood or pus.

**Treatment** The condition usually responds to antibiotics and simple painkillers. If the condition becomes chronic, patients need the specialist care of urologists and possibly a pain management clinic.

▶ *See also energy, natural therapies*

## Orchitis

A virus, such as mumps, can cause inflammation of the testes known as orchitis. Pain is severe and often accompanied by fever.

**Treatment** Inflammation and pain can be eased with painkillers and by applying icepacks to the testes. Alternating warm and cold sitz baths may also be beneficial. If the pain persists in spite of treatment, medical advice must be sought to exclude the possibility of torsion of the testicle (see page 122).

▶ *See also energy, natural therapies*

### PROSTATE PROBLEMS

Pain in the lower abdomen in men may be due to disorders of the prostate. Situated under the bladder and in front of the rectum, the gland produces some of the secretions in seminal fluid. The prostate may become inflamed, enlarged or cancerous.

## Inflamed prostate

The prostate can become inflamed, causing increased frequency of urination, pain on passing urine and sometimes difficulty. This condition is called prostatitis and is usually caused by a bacterial infection spreading from the urethra. The urine may be cloudy, and ejaculation is also often painful.

**Treatment** Prostatitis is usually treated with antibiotics. The condition has been linked to a zinc deficiency so eating zinc-rich foods, such as pumpkin and sunflower seeds or oatmeal, or taking zinc supplements may be helpful. Occasionally the condition does not clear up despite there being no evidence of infection. Treatment of chronic prostatitis may be difficult, requiring the expertise of a urologist and possibly a specialist pain management clinic.

▶ *See also massage, energy, natural therapies*

## Enlarged prostate

The prostate gland often enlarges from middle age onwards. In most men, this does not cause symptoms, but in some, an enlarged prostate constricts the urethra, blocking the flow of urine. Symptoms include difficulty urinating or incontinence. The bladder may also become distended, causing pain in the abdomen. Cancer of the prostate may also cause similar symptoms so it is important to consult a doctor as soon as possible if you experience any of them.

**Treatment** Mild symptoms usually do not require treatment although increasing your intake of zinc may be useful (see above). Naturopaths may try special massage via the rectum to improve the drainage of the gland and reduce the congestion. In severe cases, surgery may be necessary.

▶ *See also massage, movement, natural therapies*

---

### SOOTHING THE PROSTATE WITH YOGA

Yoga can help to improve blood circulation to the prostate and thus stimulate proper functioning of the organ. It also aids relaxation and reduces stress, which might otherwise inhibit the immune system and delay recovery. Try to make yoga a daily activity; it can be very useful to relieve stress built up during the day.

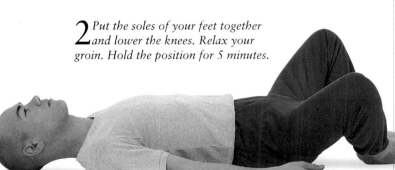

**2** *Put the soles of your feet together and lower the knees. Relax your groin. Hold the position for 5 minutes.*

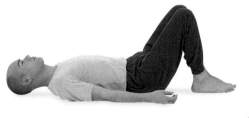

**1** *Lie on your back. You can use a blanket for support. Bend your knees, placing your feet close to your bottom.*

# MEN'S AND WOMEN'S COMPLAINTS

*Some painful, debilitating disorders of the urinary system affect both men and women. They can often be avoided by careful attention to diet and hygiene and by using safer sex practices.*

The urinary system includes the kidneys and the bladder, the tubes (ureters) connecting the kidneys to the bladder and the tube (urethra) connecting the bladder to the outside. Some urinary tract infections may be caused by sexually transmitted diseases (STDs). If an STD is left untreated, it can cause bladder and kidney infections and spread to other reproductive organs, leading to infertility. If you think you may have an STD, both you and your sexual partner should seek medical attention at once. If you prefer, your local genitourinary clinic provides advice, diagnosis and treatment in confidence and anonymously. You can reduce the risk of STDs by following safer sex practices.

### URINARY SYSTEM DISORDERS

The urinary system is susceptible to a wide variety of disorders. Although these are generally not life threatening, they can cause extreme discomfort and distress.

A burning pain when passing urine is usually due to inflammation of the bladder (cystitis) or urethra (urethritis). Infection of the bladder is more common in females – the urethra is much shorter, so infection can spread more easily. Painful urination may be a symptom of vaginal thrush (candidiasis), a sexually transmitted disease, or an allergy to perfumed soaps or deodorants.

## Kidney and ureter problems

The kidneys play an essential role in filtering the blood and removing waste products and excess water from the body. They can easily become swollen by disorders such as infections, tumours and cysts in the ureter or kidney itself. This swelling, or distension, causes extreme pain but is not generally life endangering. Kidney pain is usually felt in the lower back and there may be blood in the urine. A common problem affecting the ureter is kidney stones, which cause extreme pain as they move down the tube.

**Treatment** By caring for your kidneys you can help to prevent many of the painful conditions associated with the urinary system.

## URINARY TRACT

The urinary tract is a complex system for ridding the body of waste products. Infections of the system may affect both men and women, although urethral infections are more common in men, while bladder infections are more common in women, because of their shorter urethra.

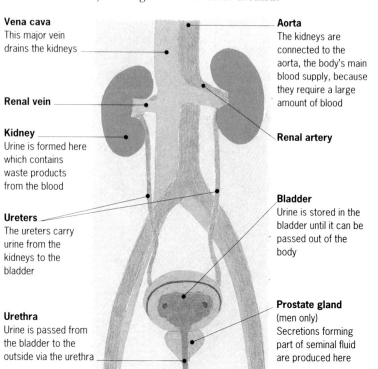

**Vena cava**
This major vein drains the kidneys

**Renal vein**

**Kidney**
Urine is formed here which contains waste products from the blood

**Ureters**
The ureters carry urine from the kidneys to the bladder

**Urethra**
Urine is passed from the bladder to the outside via the urethra

**Aorta**
The kidneys are connected to the aorta, the body's main blood supply, because they require a large amount of blood

**Renal artery**

**Bladder**
Urine is stored in the bladder until it can be passed out of the body

**Prostate gland**
(men only)
Secretions forming part of seminal fluid are produced here

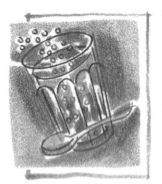

**CYSTITIS RELIEF**

Neutralising your urine can counteract the burning pain of cystitis. You can do this by eating watermelon regularly, or by mixing a teaspoon of bicarbonate of soda with a glass of water and drinking it twice a day.

**FIGHTING CYSTITIS**

Cystitis can be brought on by a variety of factors, including stress, bruising during sexual intercourse, diet, oral contraceptives, and bacteria spreading from the rectum. You can help to prevent cystitis by simple measures.

▶ *Never delay the desire to urinate.*

▶ *Always apply a lubricating jelly before intercourse.*

▶ *Try different positions if sexual intercourse brings on attacks.*

▶ *Showering and passing urine after intercourse may flush out infection.*

▶ *Wipe from front to back after going to the toilet to avoid spreading bacteria to the urethra.*

▶ *Avoid perfumed soaps, deodorants or douches that may cause irritation.*

Drinking more than 2 litres (3½ pints) of water a day helps to keep the urine diluted and thus decreases the risk of kidney stones and infection. Emptying your bladder as soon as you feel the need is also important for preventing stones from forming and bacteria from breeding. Drinking two glasses of wine a day can also reduce the risk of kidney stones developing.

▶ *See also massage, movement, natural therapies*

## Cystitis

Cystitis is an inflammation of the lining of the bladder which causes a continuous burning ache, felt deep in the pelvis. The pain may radiate to the back, lower abdomen, urethra and external genitals. Sufferers may experience painful or urgent urination, and blood in the urine. In men acute cystitis may be caused by inflammation of the prostate (see page 124).

**Treatment** Acute cystitis is best managed by drinking plenty of fluids to flush out the infection. Eat plenty of live natural yoghurt, and avoid foods that might make the urine more acidic, such as citrus fruits, tomatoes, vinegar, fish, meat and cheese. Drinking cranberry juice regularly is effective for treating and preventing urinary tract infections. Aromatherapy and herbal remedies may help to relieve the pain: add 2 drops each of essential oil of juniper berry, eucalyptus and sandalwood to a warm bath, or drink buchu tea (1 large tablespoon of leaves per cup) twice a day. If symptoms persist mild painkillers such as aspirin may help. Many people suffer recurrent attacks of cystitis – see sidebar for self-help.

▶ *See also massage, movement, energy therapies*

## Urethritis

Urethritis is inflammation of the urethra, usually due to infection. The condition can cause pain in the urethra or when passing urine, fever and an urge to urinate. Urethritis may result from a sexually transmitted disease (see page 125), a bacterial infection or, in men, an enlarged prostate.

**Treatment** The prevention and treatment of urethritis are the same as for cystitis.

▶ *See also massage, energy, natural therapies*

## Candidiasis (Thrush)

This is a fungal infection that mainly affects the vagina, although it can be passed to and from a male partner during sexual inter-

course and cause a rash on the penis. It causes soreness and intense itching of the vulva and vagina, a thick, creamy discharge and sometimes painful urination and intercourse. The *Candida albicans* microorganism that causes the condition occurs naturally in the vagina but is usually held in check by bacteria that also exist there. Anything that affects this natural balance, such as antibiotics, wearing tight clothing or using highly perfumed soaps or deodorants, can lead to infection.

**Treatment** Candidiasis is usually treated with antifungal pessaries and creams. You can often relieve the condition by applying live yoghurt to a tampon and inserting it into the vagina. Herbal, homeopathic and naturopathic remedies may also be effective.

▶ *See also massage, energy, natural therapies*

## Genital herpes

Genital herpes is a sexually transmitted disease caused by the herpes simplex virus. Common symptoms include a burning rash and multiple painful genital blisters, swollen lymph nodes, headache, fever and painful urination. Medical attention should be sought as soon as possible.

**Treatment** This condition cannot be cured but antiviral drugs may help to prevent outbreaks of blisters or make the attacks less severe. Both the severity and frequency of attacks should subside as your body builds up its own resistance. Pain may also be relieved by simple pain-relieving drugs and warm salt baths.

▶ *See also massage, energy, natural therapies*

## Chlamydia

Chlamydia is a sexually transmitted disease. In men, urination becomes painful, the testicles become swollen and often there is a discharge from the penis. Women may experience abnormal vaginal discharge, and pain during urination and sexual intercourse, but often there are no symptoms. If the condition is left untreated it can lead to pelvic inflammatory disease (see page 118). It is a major cause of infertility and miscarriage in women.

**Treatment** Chlamydia is usually treated with antibiotics. You can help to prevent chlamydia recurring by eating live yoghurt and by building up your immune system with a healthy diet.

▶ *See also massage, energy, natural therapies*

CHAPTER 8

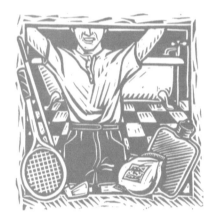

# BACK AND LIMB PAIN

---

*Probably all of us will suffer from back or limb pain to some degree at some point in our lives, yet it is poorly understood. Although in most cases medical attention is not necessary, there are some instances when these musculoskeletal pains require investigation and specific treatment. This chapter looks into a variety of types and causes of back and limb pain, and their possible treatments.*

---

# BACK AND NECK PAIN

*Back and neck pain may be caused by injury, inflammation or stress. It may also be a referred pain, due to a problem at another site away from the focus of the pain.*

Problems in the back and neck can cause severe debilitating pain. Yet in many cases examination and X-rays fail to show the cause of the pain. In addition, conventional medical techniques are unable to provide adequate relief for back and joint pain sufferers. Alternative techniques such as acupuncture and reflexology may help to ease the pain and enable you to lead a more normal life.

## DEFINING BACKACHE

Around 23 million people in Britain are said to suffer from backache. It can affect anybody at any time, regardless of age, occupation, or level of health or fitness. In most cases the pain is felt somewhere along the spine between the neck and the coccyx. This area can be divided into three sections, each of which is prone to particular kinds of pain: the lower back (lumbar sacral spine); the upper back (thoracic spine); and the neck (cervical spine).

## THE LOWER BACK

The lumbar spine, the five jointed vertebrae that make up part of the lower back, are under a lot of pressure during lifting. For this reason lower back pain, which is also known as lumbago, is most likely to affect those whose jobs involve heavy lifting or carrying. There are a wide variety of conditions that can cause lower back pain.

### Back strain

Many people experience low back pain problems after a heavy session in the garden or after working over a car engine at the weekend. Similar symptoms may be experienced after a long car or plane journey, or after sitting awkwardly for a lengthy period. The cause of these acute attacks is almost invariably back strain. In other words, you have overstretched a ligament, muscle or joint. For reasons that are poorly

## THE SPINE

The spine is the curved column of bones and cartilage extending from the base of the skull to the pelvis. Resembling a child's building blocks, the bones are supported by various ligaments, additional joints at the back, and a range of muscles both around and in front of the spine itself. In a canal behind the vertebrae is the spinal cord, an extension of the brain and vital part of the central nervous system.

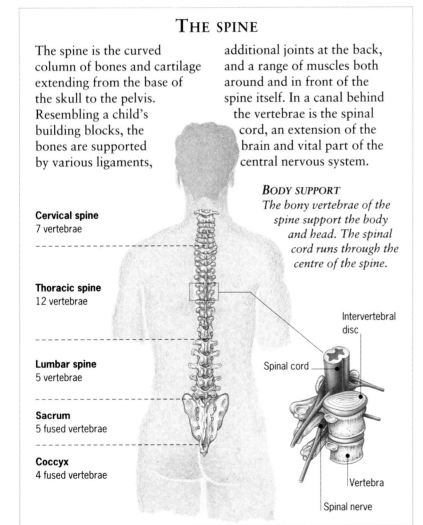

**Cervical spine**
7 vertebrae

**Thoracic spine**
12 vertebrae

**Lumbar spine**
5 vertebrae

**Sacrum**
5 fused vertebrae

**Coccyx**
4 fused vertebrae

*BODY SUPPORT*
*The bony vertebrae of the spine support the body and head. The spinal cord runs through the centre of the spine.*

Intervertebral disc

Spinal cord

Vertebra

Spinal nerve

### DID YOU KNOW?

Back pain is one of the major reasons for taking time off work. A government survey in 1996 reported that over 67 million working days in the UK are lost each year due to back pain.

understood back strain can be associated with leg pain which is similar to sciatica (see below). Unlike that condition, however, back strain is not due to pressure on a nerve. **Treatment** You can usually ease the pain of back strain with rest or by taking mild painkillers. However, too much rest can cause stiffness of the lower back which in itself creates pain as the muscles tighten and become resistant to exercise. It is therefore important to strike a happy balance between rest and activity.

If the strain recurs or becomes chronic then it is important to look at the activity that is causing it. For instance, if your work involves manual tasks such as digging or lifting, which cause pain in the lower back, specialised machinery or a more careful technique may help to overcome the potential problems. Lack of fitness and inadequate abdominal tone may cause bad posture which in turn can bring on back pain. This can be rectified by abdominal exercises or conscious improvement of your posture (see page 63).

If symptoms persist, then seek the help of a physiotherapist or other manipulative practitioner (see page 73). Ultrasound, which uses high-frequency sound to treat soft-tissue injuries, and infra-red treatment, which uses infra-red radiation, may be effective. More important, however, is to begin an exercise programme to minimise stiffness and help to prevent recurrent attacks. Pain clinics or your family GP can usually advise you on the best programme suited to your needs. Relaxation techniques can help to prevent the patient becoming depressed about the condition, which would only compound the original pain.

▶ *See also manipulative, movement, massage, energy, natural, mind, relaxation therapies*

## Disc disorders and sciatica

The spongy discs between the vertebrae consist of a soft, jelly-like core surrounded by a hard outer ring (annulus fibrosus). This outer layer is fairly elastic and is under constant pressure. In some cases the outer layer can tear, allowing the inner jelly-like material to leak into the spinal cord and put pressure on a nerve root.

This very painful condition is known as a slipped or prolapsed disc. It is usually characterised by severe lower back pain and leg pain as the nerve root is very sensitive. It is often accompanied by shooting pains and pins and needles down the leg as far as the foot. This condition is called sciatica because the pain follows the path of the sciatic nerve.

**Treatment** In most cases a slipped disc is relieved within six weeks with the aid of rest, mild painkillers and physiotherapy. However, if the pain persists over a longer period then surgery may be necessary.

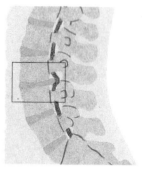

*PROLAPSED DISC*
*If a spinal disc ruptures and its soft spongy core (shown in blue) leaks out, it may put pressure on a nerve (shown in purple) causing severe pain and disability.*

## RELIEVING PAIN FROM A SLIPPED DISC

A slipped disc can respond well to simple bed rest. Lie flat on your back with your shoulders, hips and ankles aligned to ease pressure on the spine. Elevating the lower spine will also ease pressure. The exercise shown below uses two tennis balls placed in a knotted sock to raise the spine and provide relief.

*ELEVATING THE SPINE*
*Lie on the floor placing the balls under your lower back, one on either side of the spine. Hold the position for 5 minutes. Remove the balls and relax for 2 minutes, then place the balls under your buttocks and repeat the exercise.*

**Keep your knees bent** and your feet flat on the floor

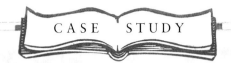
# Man with Slipped Disc

*A healthy back is remarkably resilient, able to cope with a wide range of pressures during work and leisure activities. Sudden excessive strain, however, especially if coupled with overweight and reduced flexibility due to lack of exercise, can lead to painful back injuries. In this situation, changes in diet, lifestyle and work practices may be necessary to correct the problem.*

Eric is a 32-year-old builder's labourer who works on a demolition site. Though he keeps active with football at the weekends, a taste for fry-up breakfasts and fish and chips at least twice a week have left him a few kilos overweight. One day at work Eric was wheeling a heavy wheelbarrow of bricks across the site and he suddenly felt the most excruciating pain in his back which left him unable to work for the rest of the day. A dull, intermittent pain radiated into his leg. His doctor diagnosed a prolapsed intervertebral disc and referred him to a chiropractor. Eric finds the pain unendurable and a threat to his livelihood, as he is afraid to try any activity which may aggravate it.

## WHAT SHOULD ERIC DO?

Eric should see the chiropractor for treatment, including manipulation of his spine. This treatment will help to ease the pressure on the disc by relaxing the surrounding muscles, relieving inflamed ligaments and separating the vertebral spaces. He could also try a course of acupuncture, which can relieve some of the acute pain and muscle spasm. Eric has been advised to get plenty of bed rest and he finds it takes the pressure off his back. Eric should also join a back pain association which can tell him how his back pain came about in the first place. The association will also give him tips on how to cope with his condition and avoid similar problems occurring in the future.

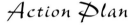

## Action Plan

**DIET**
*Replacing fatty foods with complex carbohydrates – bread and pasta, for example – will result in an eventual loss of weight without feeling low in energy.*

**LIFESTYLE**
*Cut out football. Regular stretches, and aerobic exercise such as swimming, will help to strengthen the spine. Allow time for warm-up exercises before doing physical activities.*

**WORK**
*Employ safe lifting and carrying techniques so that the back is not strained.*

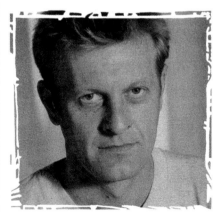

**DIET**
*Fast food in the long term is poor in nutritional value and high in fat and cholesterol.*

**LIFESTYLE**
*Being overweight increases pressure on the intervertebral discs, and potentially dangerous body contact sports such as football put further strain on the body.*

**WORK**
*Physically demanding labour can place strong pressure on the body, and the back in particular.*

## HOW THINGS TURNED OUT FOR ERIC

Eric found that several sessions of acupuncture and a course of chiropractic treatment relieved his back pain effectively. The programme of stretches and exercises that specialists taught him are also proving beneficial. He swims once or twice a week and eats healthier meals. He is losing weight at a steady rate and as he now feels much better this encourages him to carry on watching his weight. The back pain association is providing useful advice.

Placing an ice pack, wrapped in a towel, and hot-water bottle alternately on the site of the pain for 10 minutes twice a day can help to reduce sciatic pain.

▶ *See also manipulative, movement, massage, energy, natural, relaxation therapies*

### Arthritis of the spine

Discs naturally dry out and become narrower with age and this can cause chronic back pain, with or without leg pain. If the disc exerts pressure on a nerve, the back pain can be accompanied by acute attacks of sciatica. As the disc becomes narrower the facet joints behind the spine change shape and alignment and they too become worn. If this process continues, arthritis can develop, causing chronic pain and stiffness. In some people the condition may lead to narrowing of the spinal canal (spinal stenosis), which causes leg pain on walking and limits activity significantly.

**Treatment** People with arthritic spines usually have to restrict their activities as exercise, bending, stretching and lifting cause flare-ups. This may mean changing jobs. Back supports have been prescribed in the past but if worn for more than a day or so during an acute attack, they can compound the problem by weakening and stiffening the back. A balanced approach with rest, anti-inflammatory drugs and an exercise programme is the best form of treatment under these circumstances and a pain clinic (see page 69) or your GP can advise.

A natural alternative to orthodox anti-inflammatory drugs is a tincture consisting of equal parts of meadowsweet, willow bark, black cohosh, prickly ash, celery seed and nettle taken three times a day in half teaspoon amounts. To prevent stiffness try drinking aloe vera juice or applying aloe vera gel to the affected areas. Rolfing (see page 72) may help many arthritis sufferers. The founder of this technique, Ida Rolf, discovered that exercising the body's connective tissues helped to cure her own arthritis.

▶ *See also manipulative, movement, massage, energy, natural, relaxation therapies*

### Osteoporosis

As the body ages, the bones naturally become thinner. In the condition known as osteoporosis the density of the bones decreases, making them brittle and less capable of withstanding stress. Women are particularly vulnerable to this condition after the menopause when the ovaries cease producing the hormone oestrogen, which helps to maintain bone density. Osteoporosis can cause minute fractures in the vertebrae, which leads in turn to ligament and muscle strains as the overall posture of the spine is changed. Eventually the vertebrae may collapse completely, causing severe localised pain and tenderness.

**Treatment** It is difficult to replace bone tissue once it has been lost. However, it is possible to reduce the risk of osteoporosis by exercising regularly and by maintaining a balanced diet including plenty of foodstuffs containing vitamin D and calcium. A patient who lies in bed loses muscle bulk and bone mass. Walking, running, aerobics and weight-bearing exercise are all good for

## EXERCISES FOR BACKACHE

Backache is one of the most common forms of chronic pain. Regular light exercise helps to keep the muscles working efficiently and the joints supple. Develop a daily exercise programme to meet your needs together with your GP. Even if your mobility is severely limited, the exercise below can promote flexibility and relieve pain.

1 *Sit with your right leg straight out. Bend your left knee and place your left foot on the outside of your right knee.*

2 *Bend your right elbow and put it on the outside of your left thigh just above the knee. Breathe in deeply and try to straighten your back.*

3 *With your left hand behind you, slowly twist your upper body and head to look over your left shoulder. Hold for 20 seconds and repeat for the other side.*

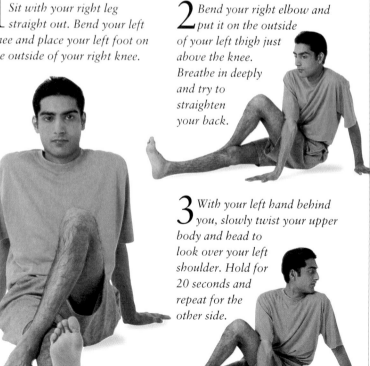

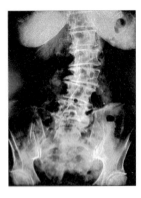

*AGE AND THE SPINE*
*The X-ray above of an elderly woman shows the characteristics of an advanced form of osteoarthritis: curvature of the spine and reduction of space between vertebrae. Increasing your intake of calcium can do much to prevent the onset of the disease. Good sources of calcium include low fat milk, yoghurt, tinned sardines and anchovies, green leafy vegetables, and beans and pulses.*

helping to minimise the loss of bone mass. Hydrotherapy exercises in hospital pools specially heated to body temperature 37°C (98.6°F) may also be effective. Provided a balanced diet is followed, supplements should not be necessary. New drug therapies are being developed but although the early results are promising they are as yet unproven. The following herbs used alone or in combination may be effective for treating oestrogen deficiencies: liquorice, black cohosh, fennel and unicorn root.
▶ *See also manipulative, movement, massage, energy, natural, relaxation therapies*

## Ankylosing spondylitis

In ankylosing spondylitis the joints between the vertebrae and the joints between the spine and the pelvis become inflamed, causing pain and stiffness in the lower back. Symptoms tend to be worse early in the morning and in some cases the stiffness may affect daily activities. The condition predominantly affects young males and tends to run in families. The condition can be treated and most sufferers are able to lead a normal life. A form of the disorder has been linked to the skin disorder psoriasis or colitis, an inflammatory disorder affecting the colon (lower bowel).

**Treatment** Pain and stiffness caused by ankylosing spondylitis may be minimised by heat therapy, massage, breathing exercises, posture training, stringent exercise programmes – including daily swimming – and non-steroidal anti-inflammatory drugs. Because of the connection with colitis in some people (see page 111), making changes to your diet may help to prevent the onset of the condition. A low-fat, low-starch and low-sugar diet may help to starve and limit the growth of undesirable bacteria. To relieve the aching and stiffness try a few drops of arnica tincture in your bath. Stretching exercises can help to prevent curvature of the spine.
▶ *See also movement, energy, natural therapies*

## Back pain in pregnancy

In the last months of pregnancy women are prone to low back problems. The increased weight of the foetus places greater strain on the muscles and ligaments of the lower back, causing pain. The pain may also be due to hormone imbalance or gynaecological complications such as a retroverted uterus. However, the pain almost always subsides after the birth.

**Treatment** Careful antenatal screening and advice on posture and suitable activities can help to minimise back pain in pregnancy. Swimming is an ideal exercise right up until the later stages of a pregnancy as the body is supported by the water, which eases the strain on weight-bearing joints. Massage is extremely beneficial for relieving back and neck pain.

### THE UPPER BACK

Back pain in the thoracic spine is usually due to damage through physical activity, such as strains in the latissimus dorsi muscle caused by lifting accidents. In the elderly, upper back pain may be due to osteoporosis. Pain may also be referred from another site; for instance, duodenal ulcers or gallstones can cause aching in the upper back.

### THE NECK

The neck is an extremely delicate structure and is thus vulnerable to several painful disorders. A patient may suffer greatly from any swelling or inflammation of the muscles or joints in the neck because they are so tightly packed together.

## Acute neck strain

If you sit over a book or keyboard for a lengthy period of time without a rest then acute neck strain may arise. A change in

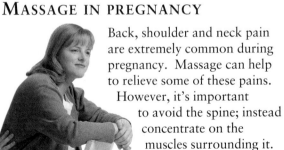

## MASSAGE IN PREGNANCY

Back, shoulder and neck pain are extremely common during pregnancy. Massage can help to relieve some of these pains. However, it's important to avoid the spine; instead concentrate on the muscles surrounding it.

*SOOTHING AN ACHING BACK*
*Sit so that you are leaning over the back of a chair. Your partner should use long sweeping strokes starting from the base of the spine and gradually moving upwards and outwards.*

position or work habits can help to prevent or treat this problem. As in the lower back, the problem never leads to arthritis.

**Treatment** Simple stretches are useful for preventing neck strain. Clasp your hands together and cup them over the back of your head. Drop your head forward and feel your neck stretching. Using one hand, push your head to one side and then do the same in the opposite direction. Taking anti-inflammatory painkillers or infusions of valerian may help to ease the pain. Compresses of an anti-inflammatory herb such as willow bark can help to relax stiff muscles. You could also try pressing on acupressure points at the top of the shoulders, a few inches out from the base of the neck, to ease the pain and stiffness.

▶ *See also manipulative, movement, massage, energy, natural, relaxation therapies*

## Whiplash injury

In a rear or head-on collision in a car, the body may be held rigid by the seat belt while the head is thrown backwards and forwards by the impact. This may cause the onset of whiplash, which is felt as an acute neck strain a few hours or even a few days after the incident. Head restraints on car seats prevent damage to the cervical spine in collisions, but must be at the appropriate level. Severe injuries, including fractures and dislocations, tend to occur only in the most violent high-speed collisions.

**Treatment** Immediately after a whiplash injury, an ice pack should be held against the painful area for 10 minutes. Then apply a hot-water bottle wrapped in a towel for another 10 minutes. Alternate these several times every morning and evening. After the initial shock of the collision has subsided, the pain usually settles but if it does not then treatment from a manipulation therapist should be sought (see page 70).

The muscles around the spinal column are very strong and support the head on the neck for all activities. For this reason after a whiplash injury surgical collars should be worn only if there is a risk of instability, as they weaken the muscles and cause further pain and stiffness. However, soft foam collars can be worn at night as this is the time when the muscles of the head and neck are relaxed. The essential oils of rosemary and sweet marjoram can relieve pain – add 2 drops of each to your bath, or to 2 teaspoons of carrier oil and rub in night and morning. Simple painkillers may also be effective. Symptoms usually ease within two to three weeks – sticking to your rehabilitation schedule is essential to prevent the development of chronic symptoms.

▶ *See also manipulative, movement therapies*

## Cervical spondylosis

Cervical spondylosis, or neck arthritis, affects the joints between the vertebrae in the neck. The discs gradually lose fluid after early middle age and become narrower. This causes pain and stiffness in the neck and numbness and tingling in the arms and hands if the disc puts pressure on the nerves. The condition occurs in the vast majority of people, but most never suffer from neck pain. However, certain individuals may be prone to the condition – manual workers, rugby players and people with other joint disorders such as rheumatoid arthritis can develop symptoms. It may also be brought on by injury, such as whiplash neck injury after a car accident.

**Treatment** Usually the pain can be controlled with simple painkillers, a collar for night wear and occasional physiotherapy, particularly if the discs are pressing on a nerve. If the condition persists then surgery may be necessary to relieve the pressure on the nerve by fusing the two problem vertebrae with a bone graft.

▶ *See also manipulative, massage therapies*

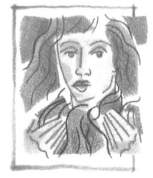

**RELAXING THE NECK**

If your neck feels tense and uncomfortable, try swathing it in a silk scarf. The warmth that this brings can help to improve blood circulation and relieve muscle pain and tension in the neck.

---

## REFLEXOLOGY FOR NECK PAIN

If your neck is too sensitive to touch, let alone massage, it may help to try massaging the feet instead. According to reflexologists, areas on the feet called reflex zones correspond to other parts of the body. If one of these zones is massaged it can relieve pain in a corresponding area of the body. You can give yourself a simple massage to relieve neck pain, but for a longer course of treatment it is advisable to contact a qualified practitioner.

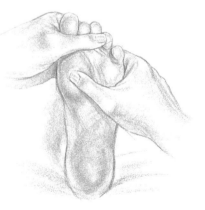

*MASSAGE FOR NECK PAIN*
*Massaging the ball of the foot and the area where the big toe joins the feet on the bottom of the foot can help to bring relief from neck pain.*

# GENERAL JOINT PAIN

*Pain in the limbs may be due to conditions arising in the joints of the arms or legs, or a referred pain from the back or neck, or it may be a symptom of a more general disorder.*

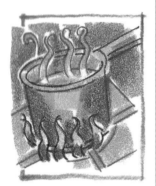

**JOINT RELIEF**

Once the swelling of painful joints has subsided, a hot compress or the following mixture can help to soothe the aches.

▶ *Boil a tablespoon of cayenne pepper with a pint of cider vinegar for 10 minutes, and allow to cool. Massage olive oil into the skin before applying to prevent skin irritation.*

▶ *Soak a clean towel with the mixture and wrap around the affected joint until the pain eases.*

There are many disorders that can cause severe pain in the limbs. In some cases, the disorder may affect a single joint such as the knee, while in other cases, several joints such as the hips, wrists and toes may be affected.

## Osteoarthritis

Osteoarthritis is a common disease of the joints causing pain, inflammation and stiffness. It is thought to be caused by a disorder of the cartilage that covers the surface of the joint. Under normal circumstances this tough and well-lubricated cartilage enables smooth movement of the joint. However, the cartilage may soften and begin to break up into flakes, some of which can form loose bodies in the joint. This causes the lining of the joint (synovium) to become inflamed and the joint to swell with excess fluid. As the cartilage breaks up, the underlying bone becomes exposed, which causes spasm, then stiffness as the patient tries to protect the diseased joint. New cartilage may be formed but this is usually of poor quality and can cause osteophytes, or overgrowths of the bone, which can hinder movement even further.

The condition can occur for no particular reason or can be hereditary. Osteoarthritis of the hip is fairly common among the elderly and also among post-menopausal women with a close relative, such as a mother or a sister, suffering from the condition. It can be brought on by other disorders such as injury or a deformity of the joint, in which case it is known as secondary osteoarthritis. **Treatment** In the early stages of the condition, non-steroidal anti-inflammatory drugs, heat (for example, a warm bath) and weight loss are effective for easing pain. If there is a large build-up of fluid in the joint, ice packs may help to reduce the inflammation. If the swelling persists, a doctor may decide to draw the fluid off with a needle and syringe. It is important to keep active and to keep the joint as mobile as possible – resting too much can cause more stiffness and affect the joint's function, for example, stiff knees can make climbing the stairs seem an impossible task.

Chiropractic and acupuncture can be effective at relieving joint pain, particularly if the osteoarthritic symptoms are caused by misalignment of the joints. You can also try massaging the muscles around the inflamed joints with your fingertips or the heel of your hand, moving with smooth and gentle strokes in the direction of the heart.

If the arthritis is too severe and does not respond to treatment then surgery may need to be considered.

▶ *See also manipulative, movement, massage, energy, natural therapies*

## Rheumatoid arthritis

Rheumatoid arthritis is a painful disorder that is characterised by inflammation and sometimes severe deformity of the joints, particularly the fingers, wrists, knees and hips. The condition is known as an autoimmune disorder in which the immune system attacks the body's own tissues for no known reason. In this case the synovial tissue lining the joints is attacked, causing inflammation. It can also affect the tendons and surrounding tissues, including the muscles and ligaments.

The most common early symptoms are stiffness in the joints of the fingers, hands or even the feet, especially in the morning. In some cases the condition may affect only one or two joints, but in others it may spread to almost all the joints in the body. Rheumatoid arthritis can affect anyone, including babies, young children and elderly people, although it most often occurs in middle-aged women.

**Treatment** Keeping the joints mobile tends to help in the early stages of the disorder. However, as time goes on, other joints may become involved, making activity more painful. Treatment of the pain is similar to that for osteoarthritis, and physiotherapists and other manipulation therapists can help considerably. Occupational therapists can advise patients on how to cope with disability and introduce devices such as special bottle openers and cutlery designed for patients with finger joint disorders.

Anti-inflammatory painkillers, such as aspirin or ibuprofen, can ease the symptoms, or try a decoction or tablets containing the anti-inflammatory devil's claw. Add 1 teaspoon of devil's claw per cupful of water, and simmer for 15 minutes. Strain and drink three times a day. To relieve the stiffness caused by rheumatoid arthritis try a cold compress. Moisten some cotton wool with cold water and wrap it around the painful joint. Cover it with two layers of flannel or wool and leave it in position for 4-8 hours. The compress should warm up within 15 minutes.

▶ *See also manipulative, movement, massage, energy, natural therapies*

## Gout

Gout is a joint disease predominantly affecting men. The big toe joint is usually affected but other joints such as the ankles, wrists and knees can be involved. The disorder is caused by a build-up of the waste product uric acid in the blood. Crystals of uric acid form within the joint, causing acute inflammation which usually lasts from seven to ten days. The affected joint becomes swollen, very tender and hot and may be accompanied by a light fever. Secondary arthritis of the affected joint may also develop.

**Treatment** Elevating the affected joint and rest are essential in the treatment of gout. Applying an ice pack for 3-5 minutes at regular intervals may help to ease the inflammation caused by an acute attack. If a large joint is affected, your doctor may decide to remove excess fluid with a needle and syringe. In some cases tablets which help to reduce the level of uric acid in the blood may be prescribed. As uric acid levels may be increased by high levels of a substance known as purine, avoiding foods high in purine, such as liver, poultry and pulses (see below), may help to reduce the risk of suffering future attacks.

According to some naturopaths eating celery seed helps to eliminate excess uric acid in the blood. You can make an infusion by pouring boiling water onto 2 teaspoons of crushed seeds. Allow the mixture to steep for 15 minutes and then drink a cupful three times a day. Cutting down on alcohol and losing weight may also help to prevent the frequency of acute gout attacks.

▶ *See also manipulative, movement, massage, energy, natural therapies*

**Cure from the sea**
A simple marine creature called the sea cucumber may offer hope for osteoarthritis sufferers. According to a 1993 study by the University of Queensland in Australia, eating sea cucumbers can help to alleviate the pain of osteoarthritis because they contain chemical agents which attack the disease. After successful trials at the university, the Australian Department of Health authorised the use of the active ingredients isolated from sea cucumbers as an arthritis treatment.

## FIGHTING GOUT

Naturopaths believe that a change of diet can help to reduce the risk of recurring attacks of gout. They suggest you eat more foods that tend to lower the amount of uric acid in the blood and avoid those foods that tend to raise it.

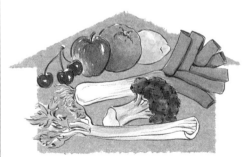

*FOODS TO FIGHT GOUT*
Eat cherries and other berries, apples, citrus fruits such as oranges and lemons, and vegetables such as leeks, broccoli and celery.

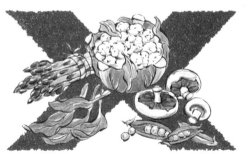

*GOUT-CAUSING FOODS TO AVOID*
Stay away from peas and pulses, mushrooms, cauliflower, asparagus and spinach. Also avoid red meat, shellfish, poultry and offal.

**Nightshade**
An arthritis specialist in the United States, Dr Robert Bingham, found that a third of his rheumatoid arthritis patients were sensitive to plants of the nightshade family, such as potatoes, tomatoes, peppers, avocados and tobacco. To test whether they are contributing to your arthritic pain you can try eliminating these foods from your diet.

# PROBLEMS AFFECTING SPECIFIC JOINTS

*Joints may be affected by inflammation of surrounding tissues such as tendons. Rest and manipulative treatments can help to ease the pain, but occasionally, surgery may be necessary.*

Two of the most common conditions affecting specific joints are inflammation of the tendons (tendinitis) and inflammation of the bursa (bursitis). The bursa are fluid-filled pads that act as shock absorbers at joints such as the shoulder, elbow, knee and wrist.

### THE SHOULDER

The shoulder is an extremely complicated joint. Pain can arise for a variety of reasons. Arthritis is most likely to be associated with disorders such as rheumatoid arthritis or a previous injury, for example from playing sport or through occupational damage.

## Tendinitis and bursitis

Many painful shoulder disorders are caused by problems in the subacromial space, just above the shoulder joint and below the collarbone, or clavicle. This space houses a tendon and a bursa, a pad that acts as a buffer and lubricates it to enable smooth movement. The tendon may be injured, or the bursa can become inflamed. Both problems cause pain when the arm is raised.

**Treatment** Applying an ice pack to the area for 30 minutes three to four times a day for the first 48 hours may ease the pain. After two days, apply moist heat with a poultice, hot pack or hot shower for 20 minutes at a time, several times a day. Use gentle exercise to restore movement by swinging the arm gently and loosely. As soon as you can, begin to raise both arms over your head several times a day, reaching higher each day. It may help to visualise the pain as a sword in the joint. Imagine that ice is applied to the site and the sword is gradually drawn out; feel the pain gradually decreasing. If symptoms persist, the doctor may suggest corticosteroid injections.
▶ *See also manipulative, movement therapies*

## Arthritis of the shoulder joint

Where the collarbone meets the shoulder blade there is a flat joint, the acromioclavicular joint, which moves very little. It can become arthritic, particularly in sportsmen or workers who carry loads on their shoulders, such as hod carriers.

**Treatment** Local injections into the joint can help but surgery may be necessary. Problems in the joint can cause it to press down on the subacromial space below, leading to symptoms similar to tendinitis.
▶ *See also manipulative, movement therapies*

---

## THE SHOULDER

Painful disorders affecting the shoulder are common. Problems such as bursitis can affect the shoulder joint itself and the acromioclavicular joint. The mobility of the joint may also be affected by inflamed shoulder tendons and muscles.

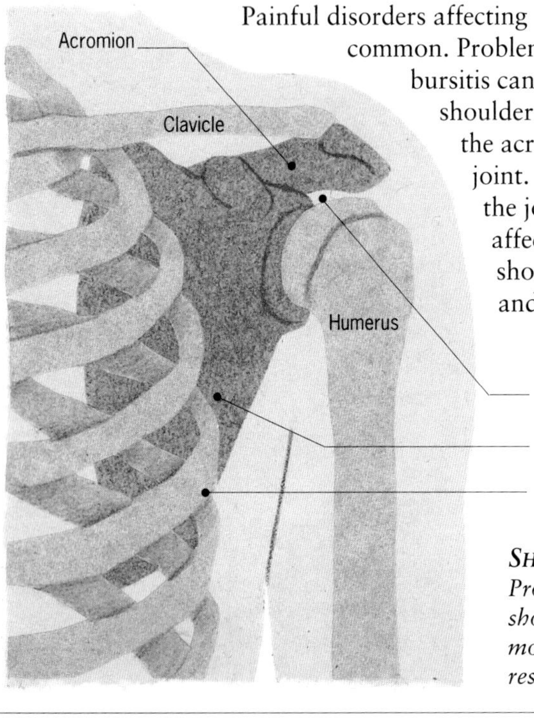

Acromion

Clavicle

Humerus

Subacromial space

Scapula

Rib cage

*SHOULDER PAIN*
*Problems in the shoulder may result in movement being restricted completely.*

## Frozen shoulder

Frozen shoulder is caused by inflammation of the lining of the joint socket. Usually the shoulder is painful to move, and in severe cases it can become very stiff. The condition particularly affects people with diabetes and those recovering from a stroke. Although the term is often used for shoulder pain, the condition is quite rare. In many cases the problem lies in the subacromial space.

**Treatment** Frequent application of ice packs and a course of very gentle but gradually progressing exercises are necessary to keep the shoulder mobile. Hydrotherapy can be very effective, and massaging the muscles of the shoulder and those extending into the chest, back and neck will help to relieve tension and encourage movement. Osteopathic or chiropractic treatment can help to ease the pain and restore mobility. Acupuncture may also be effective.

▶ *See also manipulative, massage therapies*

### THE ELBOW

Several painful disorders can affect the elbow, including arthritis and injuries to the joint and the surrounding muscles, ligaments and tendons.

## Tennis elbow

Overuse of the extensor muscles on the thumb side of the elbow, which straighten the wrist and fingers, causes strain on the tendon attaching the elbow to the bone of the upper arm. The tendon can become inflamed, causing a painful condition called tennis elbow, or lateral epicondylitis. The disorder can be brought on by acute injury or by a repetitive activity such as painting a wall, keyboard work or racquet sports.

**Treatment** To reduce inflammation, rest the arm and apply ice packs for the first 24 hours. Then bathe the elbow alternately in hot and cold water or apply ice packs followed by a warm rub and brisk towel dry. This stimulates circulation and aids healing. Acupuncture and frequent massage of the affected area with essential oils of lavender or rosemary also helps to stimulate blood flow. Corticosteroids injected into the area may be effective, but if symptoms persist then other treatments such as a forearm clasp may be advised. This is particularly useful for sportsmen or manual workers. Surgery is rarely necessary.

▶ *See also manipulative, massage therapies*

## Golfer's elbow

Overuse of the flexor muscles, which bend the wrist and fingers, causes inflammation and tenderness or pain on the inner side of the elbow. The condition, medial epicondylitis, or golfer's elbow, is particularly prevalent in people who exercise frequently and in manual workers engaged in digging.

**Treatment** Golfer's elbow is best treated with rest and ice packs as for tennis elbow.

▶ *See also manipulative, movement therapies*

### THE WRIST

Wrist pain may be caused by a variety of conditions, including degenerative joint diseases, such as arthritis, and inflammation of the tendon, such as tenosynovitis.

## Carpal tunnel syndrome

The median nerve passes into the hand via a passageway called the carpal tunnel. The median nerve may get compressed within the tunnel, causing pain and numbness in the wrist or thumb and fingers. The problem can occur for no apparent reason, but pregnant women, those with an underactive thyroid gland, diabetic patients and overweight menopausal women are at increased risk. Symptoms tend to be worse at night.

**Treatment** The numbness and tingling may be relieved by shaking the wrist and hand or elevating it. Wearing a splint at night may help to soothe the pain. In severe cases surgery to relieve the pressure on the nerve may be necessary.

▶ *See also manipulative, movement, massage, energy, natural therapies*

### Acupressure points for carpal tunnel syndrome

An acupressure point that can be used to relieve wrist pain can be found in the middle of the inner forearm two and a half finger lengths above the wrist crease. Firmly press this point on the affected arm for 2 minutes and repeat three times daily for a month. Alternatively try a point the same distance above the wrist crease on the outside of the forearm between the two bones.

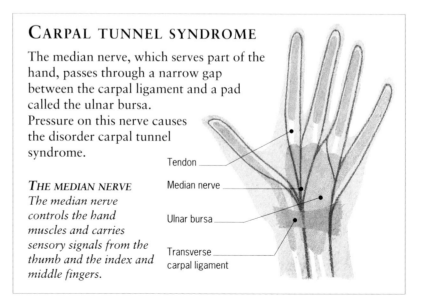

## CARPAL TUNNEL SYNDROME

The median nerve, which serves part of the hand, passes through a narrow gap between the carpal ligament and a pad called the ulnar bursa. Pressure on this nerve causes the disorder carpal tunnel syndrome.

*THE MEDIAN NERVE*
*The median nerve controls the hand muscles and carries sensory signals from the thumb and the index and middle fingers.*

Tendon

Median nerve

Ulnar bursa

Transverse carpal ligament

## Tenosynovitis

If the inner lining of the sheath surrounding a tendon becomes inflamed, for example through overuse, it can cause swelling, tenderness and even severe pain, a condition known as tenosynovitis. Usually affecting the wrist and hand, the condition is most often seen in those whose jobs involve repetitive actions, such as factory workers, typists and computer operators.

**Treatment** Wearing a splint, resting the wrist and taking anti-inflammatory drugs usually help to alleviate the pain. However, if the pain persists, corticosteroid drugs may be injected into the wrist. Surgery may be necessary if fibrous bands develop between the tendon and its sheath.

### THE KNEE

Knees are complicated joints which are prone to injury, leading to inflammation of the joints, tendons and bursas, bleeding into the joint, and arthritis.

## Sports injuries

The menisci, or crescent-shaped cartilages, in the knee, help to increase joint stability, but can tear, causing severe pain. Tendon strains and ruptures, muscle tears and tendinitis are also common injuries among active sportsmen and women.

**Treatment** Ice packs, rest and physiotherapy help to relieve acute pain. More severe injuries may require surgery.

▶ *See also manipulative, movement, massage, energy, relaxation therapies*

## Occupational knee problems

Miners and other people who work in the same position for long periods are prone to tears in the cartilage. These injuries require the same treatment as sports injuries. Kneeling on all fours for a long time, for example while fitting a carpet, can cause pre-patella bursitis, or housemaid's knee, when the bursa in front of the kneecap (patella) becomes swollen with fluid and inflamed. Kneeling in an upright position for a long period places great stress on the patella, tendon and shin area. This causes similar symptoms to housemaid's knee and is known as parson's knee.

**Treatment** If the joint is severely inflamed, apply an ice pack to the affected area three times a day (see page 155). Apply for 5 minutes, remove for 5 minutes, and then replace for another 10 minutes. Once the swelling has reduced, apply a hot compress to the knee to aid healing. Corticosteroid injections in the bursae can help to reduce the inflammation and surgery is rarely necessary. Protective kneepads can prevent the problem occurring.

▶ *See also manipulative, movement therapies*

### THE FOOT

There are a number of causes of painful feet. In some people the balls of the feet are prominent, which can be a cause of pain. In this case the problem can be managed by placing appropriate insoles in the shoes.

## Foot disorders

These include painful swellings in the nerve in the front of the foot which give rise to neuroma, or nerve swellings, which cause significant pain. This condition is known as Morton's neuroma. Occasionally a bunion, a swelling of the bursa around a big toe joint, can cause pain. Arthritis may arise in the big toe joint, which can become stiff and require wider shoes or even surgery.

**Treatment** Placing an ice pack on the painful area for 10 minutes while sitting with the leg raised may help to relieve the pain. Repeat the process every 10 minutes. If bunions result from wearing narrow high-heeled shoes, switching to roomy flat shoes can help to prevent chronic pain. Try to flex your toes whenever possible. Exercise the toes by putting an elastic band around them and trying to flex them outwards. If the condition persists, surgery may be necessary.

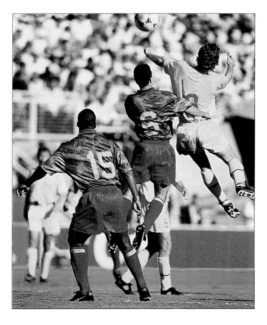

*FOOTBALL INJURIES*
*Footballers are frequently affected by knee injuries. Sports physiotherapists are specially trained to relieve the pain caused by common strains and tears.*

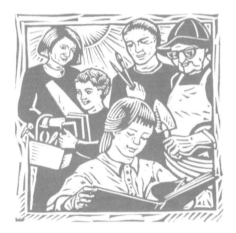

# CHAPTER 9

# LIVING WITH CHRONIC PAIN

*Sufferers of chronic painful disorders can all too easily fall into a negative cycle of depression, tension and irritability. This not only worsens the original pain but can also have serious consequences for the person's job, family and social life. Learning to live with chronic pain means breaking out of this cycle by first accepting and then mastering your pain.*

# COPING WITH PAIN

*Finding a positive way to live with chronic pain is a two-step process: the first step is to come to terms with your pain, and the second is to master it.*

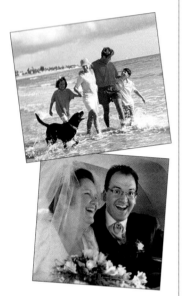

**POSITIVE IMAGERY**
*Try digging deep down into your memory to remember and relive some of the positive experiences in your life, such as pleasant family holidays, the first days of your relationship with your partner, the day you were promoted. Once you can learn to push the pain to the back of your mind and stop thinking about it, your condition and general mental health should start to improve.*

Chronic pain can affect anybody, regardless of age or sex. Chronic pain often has no purpose, unlike acute pain which serves as a distress signal to warn of injury or illness. It is often regarded as a 'useless' pain because it may persist long after an injury has healed, or it may be caused by a chronic disease or disorder, such as cancer or arthritis, long after the onset of the disease has made any 'warning' sign redundant. In some cases there may even be no apparent physical cause.

Chronic pain tends to be constant rather than intermittent so it can seriously interfere with your daily activities. In fact, the situation may seem hopeless, but an understanding of chronic pain and the way it is linked with your emotions and lifestyle really can help you to learn to rise above the condition and the problems it causes.

### SURVIVING CHRONIC PAIN

Chronic pain poses emotional and psychological problems which can be at least as damaging as the physical consequences. People who are in chronic pain suffer from a complex web of negative feelings, which in turn can affect not only the sufferer's well-being but also that of family, close friends and work colleagues.

### The unpredictability of pain

As persistent pain is unpredictable and often without apparent cause, a major worry for sufferers is feeling that they are not believed. One day the pain may stay at a manageable level and the next day – for no apparent reason – it may flare-up and force the person to take a day off work, miss a family outing or cancel a holiday. The erratic nature of chronic pain makes it hard for family, friends and colleagues to understand and sympathise. Even doctors can be confused by some cases of chronic pain as X-rays and other tests may show no signs of a disorder.

**Coping strategy** Chronic pain sufferers should realise that there may be no simple explanation for their problems. Many patients go to the doctor with their hopes raised expecting their illness to be named and an antidote prescribed, and when this fails to happen they become depressed. Instead of leaving it all up to the doctor, try taking responsibility for your health.

You should aim to find out all you can about your condition and the underlying cause of the pain – for example, knowing that pain can continue even though healing has taken place can help you to understand what is happening to your body.

You can also prepare yourself for a visit to the doctor by keeping a pain diary and marking a pain scale daily (see pages 42-45). The information gathered in this way can help to allay fears and improve communication with your doctor. Deep breathing exercises may help to release tension and focus your mind before a consultation with a doctor, and positive imagery (see left) can help to control the pain and also help to foster an optimistic outlook.

### Avoiding irritability and depression

When pain becomes so dominant in your life, it can become very wearing both for you and those around you. Constant pain, such as a sore back or an internal pain that causes nausea, can deplete energy levels and interfere with regular sleep. It can also feel

**DID YOU KNOW?**
The term 'chronic' comes from the Greek word 'khronos' which means 'time' and refers to consistent pain experienced over a long period. Aristotle, the Greek philosopher, believed pain was one of the passions of the soul, like pleasure, and that it could be conquered with reason.

humiliating if you need assistance to do things that previously you had taken for granted. The most ordinary of tasks such as getting up in the morning, dressing or climbing stairs can become an ordeal. Inevitably feelings of frustration and use-lessness, mood swings, irritability and bad temper may result.

This can lead to negative thinking: many chronic pain sufferers start to believe that their pain is a punishment and become bur-dened with guilt and bitterness. This only serves to increase the downward spiral of depression, tension and drug dependence, which worsens the sufferer's condition and quality of life.

**Coping strategy** To avoid intrusive levels of pain dominating your life, it's necessary to distract your mind. Relaxation therapies (see page 91) and visualisation exercises (see below) can all help to provide some relief, not just from pain but from the constant concern about pain. Positive thoughts can affect much more than your mind: they actually bring about physiological changes in the body because the blood flow is stimu-lated, more endorphins are released and the body functions more efficiently.

## Maintaining relationships

Family relationships are put under stress by chronic pain. The sufferer's emotional state may change on an hourly basis in response to fluctuating pain levels, which makes them unpredictable and irritable. Tension and resentment can result, especially if fam-ily members do not understand or believe the sufferer.

**Coping strategy** Communication is the key to overcoming tension between you and your family and friends. Try to explain your experience of pain as clearly as possible, describing its pattern (or its unpredictabil-ity) and intensity. In this way family and friends come to a better understanding of the nature of your pain and find it easier to accept that it exists when you say it does. You may find that family counselling is helpful at this difficult period.

Pain clinics and self-help organisations can introduce you to counsellors who can advise you and your family individually or together on these issues. Family members in particular need to know how to strike a balance between giving adequate support and allowing the chronic pain sufferer to become increasingly dependent.

### GOING BACK TO WORK

Losing your job through illness can have a huge impact on your self-esteem, causing depression and feelings of uselessness. If you're absent from work for a long period, it may be difficult to summon up the enthusiasm and confidence to return to your job. Take the following steps to readjust to working life:

▶ *Accept that your condition may require a reappraisal of your current employment. You may only be able to work part-time, for example, or you may consider retraining for another position.*

▶ *In the weeks preceding your return to work, try to increase your level of mobility. Set daily targets for exercise, such as walking a little farther every day.*

▶ *Accept the new limitations: compare your efforts with your performance when you were at your lowest ebb rather than your abilities before you fell ill.*

▶ *Once back at work, don't overdo it but build up gradually until you approach your former levels of activity.*

---

## TAKING CHARGE OF YOUR BRAIN

Visualisation exercises can help to ease stress and tension and in turn lessen the degree of pain you experience.
A particularly effective visualisation could be imagining yourself walking through your own mind, taking charge of emotions, memories and the pain sensation itself. Picture yourself as the engineer in charge of your brain, prioritising positive thoughts and memories and consigning negative thoughts to the waste bin.

*MIND POWER*
*Recent research has shown that positive thoughts actually bring about physiological changes such as increased blood flow.*

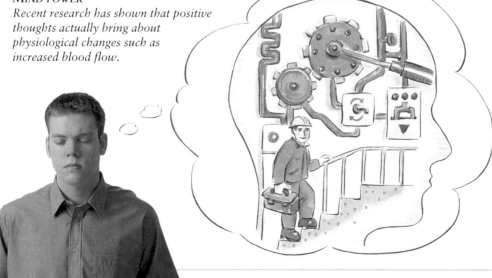

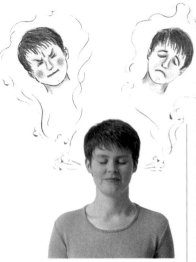

***BREATHING EXERCISE***
*Building up a relaxation programme will help you to push pain to the back of your mind. Eventually you will find you feel calmer for increasingly longer periods of the day. Breathe deeply from your diaphragm, and each time you breathe out, tell yourself that you are releasing all of your anger and sadness.*

## Readjusting at work

Chronic pain can make a demanding job much more difficult. The physical symptoms of your pain can pose very real problems in the work place; for example, back and neck pain can be exacerbated not just by physically taxing jobs but also by immobility, such as sitting at a desk for long periods. Psychological factors are equally important. Chronic pain may diminish your sense of autonomy in your job and your self-esteem and confidence in turn may be lessened.

**Coping strategy** It is important for your psychological health to try to keep working in some capacity, to give you a sense of independence and purpose, to maintain social contacts and to refocus your mind away from your pain. Many employers are now more sympathetic to chronic pain. Discuss the implications of your condition with your manager and talk about options for part-time or less demanding duties.

## Lifestyle changes

The impact of chronic pain on your lifestyle depends on its nature and severity. Many sufferers find that their favourite leisure activities such as playing sport, and even their basic mobility is seriously affected by pain. Boredom and frustration can be very real problems if you're unable to keep active and busy. Your sense of independence and self-worth can be adversely affected if you find you are dependent on others for many things previously taken for granted.

**Coping strategy** Housework, DIY, further education, hobbies, shopping and socialising do not have to disappear altogether, they simply need to be approached at a more relaxed pace and with adequate rest periods. The most important factor is to remain active. Even if you're not able to work, there's no reason why you should have to give up hobbies and interests.

Doing something creative, such as growing house plants or painting, can help to distract you from your pain and raise your self-esteem. You can also learn a great deal from other sufferers. Many pain clinics offer the opportunity to meet fellow sufferers with whom you can share problems and work together to find lifestyle solutions.

## Being in control of your pain

Perhaps the most important management technique to acquire is the ability to accept chronic pain in your life, and to be realistic about your capabilities. While positive thoughts are helpful in relieving depression, having expectations that are too high can lead to great disappointment. Become well informed about the nature of your pain, its mechanisms, and the exercises and therapies that you can undertake; the key is to feel in control of your pain.

## THE REP PROGRAMME

There are three key principles to managing your own pain effectively: relaxation, exercise and pacing – the REP programme. Balancing these three elements on a daily basis will bring real dividends. Practise relaxation methods such as deep breathing and autogenic training to help to overcome depression and negative mind-sets. Relaxation can also be very valuable after exercise to soothe any pain problems. Use exercise to combat muscle tension and relieve stress; and pace yourself both to avoid overstrain and to measure progress. For example, use a pain journal to plot exercise goals and achievements on a daily or weekly basis.

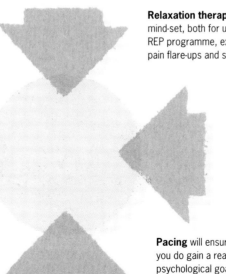

**Relaxation therapies** can establish a positive mind-set, both for undertaking the next stage of the REP programme, exercise, and dealing with existing pain flare-ups and stress.

**Exercise** will relieve muscle tension and improve mobility. Increased independence of movement will also lift your mood, and stimulate the body's own painkillers, endorphins.

**Pacing** will ensure you never overstrain yourself, but that you do gain a real sense of progress as physical and psychological goals are reached. Even setting the smallest of goals, such as extending a walk by an extra 3 minutes a day, provides long-term results.

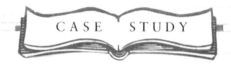
# Chronic Pain Sufferer

*Chronic pain not only affects the sufferer but can also put a strain on relatives and close friends, who may need to show great patience and tolerance. To manage chronic pain effectively requires finding a new approach to the problem, including measures such as counselling and relaxation therapies, and the active support of the whole family.*

Jane is 41 years old, married to John and with two children aged 12 and 6. A former nurse, she injured her back at work two years ago and was diagnosed as having a prolapsed disc. She now has persistent pain, which prevents her from sitting for long periods, and she cannot walk far. Although her doctor prescribes painkillers, she finds that these make her feel lethargic and irritable and tries to avoid taking them as much as possible. She can perform few tasks around the house, spends most of the day in bed, sleeps badly and feels angry that she can no longer look after her family. Her family, who now take on all the domestic chores, feel very distressed about her pain but are unsure how to help.

## WHAT SHOULD JANE DO?

Jane should ask for a referral to her local pain clinic. Initially she will attend weekly sessions with a pain management psychologist and a physiotherapist. The pain specialists will also review her medication. They can provide details of helpful booklets and tapes and put her in touch with a self-help group where she can learn relaxation techniques to help her to cope with the stress of chronic pain. The consultants will suggest a weekly family conference to discuss existing problems and help them to understand Jane's new self-help approach. An occupational therapist will visit the home in order to assess the possible introduction of useful equipment and to advise on necessary adaptations.

## Action Plan

### THE FAMILY
*Take charge of pain management rather than feeling dependent on others. Encourage the family to be patient and to allow her to cope as best she can on her own.*

### STRESS
*Practise daily relaxation strategies to cope with stress and work through problems one-by-one.*

### EMOTIONAL HEALTH
*Counselling can help to confront the wider implications of pain and its long-term effect on the family. A weekly conference will let the family discuss practical and emotional issues.*

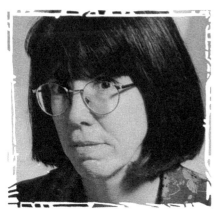

### THE FAMILY
*Jane's family are overprotective and do everything for her. They also let her indulge in too much pain talk and behaviour.*

### EMOTIONAL HEALTH
*Jane is depressed and bitter about her losses: her career, her lack of mobility, and the feeling that she is letting down her family by no longer being able to care for them adequately.*

### STRESS
*Jane's pain causes health, money, marital and family tensions that add extra strains.*

## HOW THINGS TURNED OUT FOR JANE

Jane learnt more about chronic pain and began to appreciate the possibilities for self-help. Listening to her family at the weekly conference made Jane realise how much they too were suffering, and motivated her to work at her self-help pain management. She practises relaxation exercises regularly and finds that these help her to deal more effectively with pain, and she has been able to become more active about the house.

# CARING FOR PEOPLE IN CHRONIC PAIN

*Caring for someone who suffers from chronic pain means trying to find a balance between providing support and love on the one hand, and allowing independence and self-help on the other.*

Every sufferer of chronic pain has unique care requirements and the nature of the care they need is determined by a range of factors. In each case there is a different pattern of pain, so that sufferers will lie at different points along a spectrum of disability. At one end are those who are effectively crippled by pain. At the other end there are people who need moral support and practical help when they suffer an occasional 'flare-up', but are otherwise physically fit, mobile and functioning well in all areas of their life. Nonetheless, common principles apply in all cases, whether a sufferer is old or young, able or bedridden.

### LEARNING TO PROVIDE CARE

Being a carer poses many problems. People who are close to someone with chronic pain can feel helpless and even guilty for being healthy. On the other hand they may grow to resent the attention that the sufferer demands – and then feel guilty about that.

In fact the most useful role for the carer may be to relieve one of a sufferer's major frustrations – having to continually explain their illness. People in chronic pain frequently report that trying to educate others about the quirks caused by their 'invisible' disability – without wanting to relinquish their independence or cause a fuss – can be a major difficulty. By acting as an intermediary and taking on the burden of explanation a carer can relieve this pressure, and in so doing help to remove the pain from centre stage.

The carer should try to become familiar with the particular pattern of pain that their friend or loved one experiences. Are there any triggers which spark off the pain

or things which help to soothe it? Does it follow a daily pattern? How much can the sufferer manage at any one time? By knowing these facts the carer can plan to help when severe bouts occur, affecting the sufferer's concentration or mobility, and help to protect the sufferer against triggers without having to be overprotective generally.

### Giving round-the-clock care

While emotional and social support may be all that some sufferers require, others will need help with difficult or personal tasks. Some may even need round-the-clock care and intensive nursing. These people are at particular risk of becoming invalids. Until recently, for example, it was common practice for bed rest to be prescribed for people with severe chronic back pain – for months and even years. This is now known to be a cause of muscle wasting – as much as 3 per cent of muscles can be wasted per day – and general weakness. Experts in the field now acknowledge that, except for a small minority who are seriously disabled, enforced immobility and inactivity causes more pain in the long run.

In most chronic pain cases, current practice now favours active, gentle mobilisation and early physical therapy rehabilitation. People in chronic pain are encouraged to do as much as they can, within sensible and humane parameters, for themselves. Carers are persuaded to stand gently back and allow sufferers to care for themselves as much as possible and in their own time.

Where it is necessary to provide day-to-day 24-hour care it is important that client and carer ask for a 'medical team case conference' with their doctor, nurse, psychologist, physiotherapist and any other essential

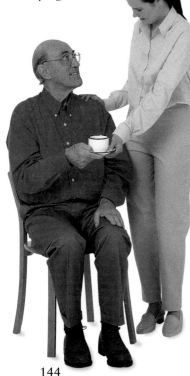

healthcare agents. This will help to establish a clear-cut rehabilitation plan and is an opportunity to ask about any local and national support organisations. Carers should also make sure to ask about the financial and personnel support they are entitled to.

## Taking care of yourself

Both caring and being cared for can exhaust good humour or worse. Failed surgery, unsuccessful treatments, poor sleep and even pain medications can cause extremes of mood. Counselling support should be accessible for the carer as well as for the patient or client. If this support is not forthcoming, carers can develop symptoms similar to post-traumatic stress, and family relationships may suffer as well. If managed properly, however, caring for someone, and being cared for, can be an enriching and enlightening experience.

### CARING FOR ELDERLY PEOPLE

Old people may feel lonely and isolated if they have outlived many of their friends and relatives, so the best care is often simply companionship and a sympathetic ear. Research shows that elderly people's experience of pain can be influenced more by environmental influences than their pain itself.

## Staying active

Keeping an elderly person mentally, socially and physically active is important – as with a sufferer of any age. Passive interests such as watching television and reading do not provide as much distraction from pain as more active pursuits like knitting, sewing and domestic chores. Teaching self-help pain management techniques or providing contact with self-help, social and recreational groups can all increase activity levels.

Another finding of research is that for many elderly people peace of mind, and thus the ability to deal with chronic pain, depends largely on how they view their past. Memories are of particular importance in old age, and good ones can be a tremendous boon to sufferers. People with regrets and bad memories, on the other hand, are more likely to feel lonely and depressed. Carers can help by encouraging their charges to discuss their memories and how they feel about them, talking them through to try to see bad memories in a positive light. Getting

sufferers to plan their memoirs, for instance, can be an excellent starting point.

Other factors also affect how an elderly person copes with pain, such as: the loss of friends and family, or financial or domestic problems. In these cases the carer should provide practical help where necessary and social support during periods of adjustment.

### CARING FOR THE TERMINALLY ILL

Terminally ill people suffering from chronic pain may falsely believe that their pain, and other common symptoms, are inevitable. In practice this is rarely the case. Pain, nausea, fatigue, constipation, loss of appetite and incontinence can all be relieved with the right help from a doctor, nurse or well-informed carer.

When the condition of a loved one or friend deteriorates and he or she becomes terminal, it is time for the carer and sufferer to reassess things together. This may be a good time to call another care conference and make a detailed care plan. It is also the time for the carer to try to prepare for the inevitable by finding out what will happen at death and afterwards.

## Putting the sufferer in control

If the sufferer is to stay on top of pain and deal with it successfully, he or she needs to retain control over their treatment plan. More specifically, putting the patient in

*COMMUNICATING PAIN*
*To help children to express pain issues, foster a positive creative atmosphere in which the problem can be discussed by all the family.*

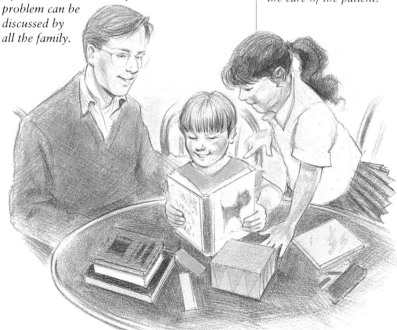

### HELPING A CHILD IN PAIN

Children feel pain just as intensely as adults – disorders such as rheumatoid arthritis and migraine can cause children to suffer from persistent pain. A parent's reaction to a child's pain can have a huge influence on the way he or she deals with pain. Parents can help their children in many ways:

▶ *Become fully informed on the latest treatment and care options.*

▶ *Ease anxiety and distress by explaining procedures and the hospital environment.*

▶ *Formulate an action plan to minimise pain levels and distress, and teach and practise skills for coping with flare-ups to reduce fear of pain.*

▶ *Incorporate visualisation, stretching and exercise, and relaxation techniques into the daily activities.*

▶ *Make sure that other siblings don't feel left out by involving them in the care of the patient.*

control of their painkilling medication has been shown to be the most effective way of cutting down on overprescription, and reducing the attendant side effects.

Keeping the person in care well informed about their condition, and involved in monitoring and assessing their own progress, also helps to reduce their anxiety and pain. Involving them in simple procedures like measuring blood pressure and temperature will help.

### CARE OPTIONS

Carers need to be aware of the options that are available for their charges. The terminally ill often need a very demanding level of 24-hour care, and there may be technical difficulties associated with medication, feeding and bowel problems that make professional help a necessity. You should attend a case conference comprising the health professionals that are treating the patient, and check out all relevant sources of information to find out what help is available.

For a terminal cancer patient, the local hospice team will supervise care for the patient and the close family. For terminal patients with non-cancer conditions, care systems will vary considerably. Normally, a district nurse will oversee care under the direction of the GP and specialists.

Community day care staff may be available, as well as night staff to come in as night-sitters – in some areas their services will be free. Private nurses are available to anyone with the financial resources to cover their fees. As it is such an exhausting and stressful time, relatives need to ask for all the quality back-up help they can get.

### Hospices

If home and hospital care options have been exhausted, the best choice may be to admit the patient to a hospice. Because of their high staff-to-patient ratio, such institutions almost always offer the best standard of care available to terminally ill people. They are not only experienced in dealing with the difficult aspects of chronic physical pain, they can also cope with the emotional and spiritual pain that the terminally ill may be facing. Staff at hospices are also well able to cope with the other symptoms that can afflict the very ill, such as pressure sores, dehydration and constipation.

A hospice provides a positive spirit and a supportive atmosphere enabling the terminally ill to come to terms with approaching death. The aim is for patients to live out their final days with a feeling of peace, calm and dignity in an environment that is free from needless pain, fear and stress.

## Origins

Dame Cicely Saunders was responsible for a major breakthrough in the management of pain when she established Saint Christopher's Hospice in south London in 1967. The hospice was not only dedicated to the care of patients, but also to research and teaching on all aspects of pain. Among her theories of pain management was that fear and anxiety directly enhanced pain by increasing tension, and that patients needed to be informed about the details of their condition in order to understand their pain and reduce their fear. She also recognised that hospices needed to provide advice to carers looking after patients at home. Saint Christopher's has since become a model for similar centres throughout the world. Her motto, adopted by the whole hospice movement, is to keep patients 'dignified, alert and pain free'.

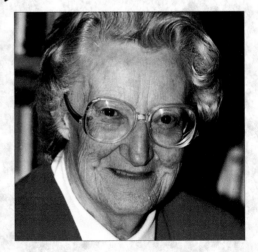

**DAME CICELY SAUNDERS**
*Dame Cicely was medical director of the first modern hospice in the UK from its establishment in 1967 until her recent retirement.*

# CHAPTER 10

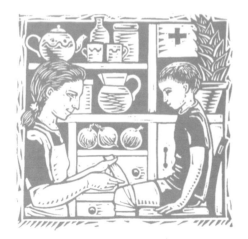

# PAIN CAUSED BY INJURIES

*The pain of minor injuries can be quickly relieved using appropriate first-aid measures and simple natural remedies that can be found in any well-stocked kitchen. In cases of more serious injuries requiring expert medical attention, prompt first aid can still ease the casualty's pain and distress and may even save a life.*

# RELIEVING THE PAIN OF MINOR INJURIES

*Accidental injuries are an ever-present threat, both indoors and out. A well-planned natural medicine cabinet and prompt first aid can provide relief from pain and ensure speedy tissue repair.*

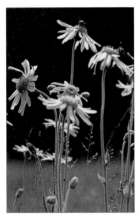

***ARNICA***
*Arnica montana, or wolfsbane, is a toxic plant with medicinal uses. The flowers contain compounds that reduce inflammation and aid circulation. It is effective as a tincture or salve for bruises, sprains and muscle pain. As the herb is toxic, it should not be applied to cuts or grazed skin or taken internally except as a homeopathic remedy (in which the ingredient is present in undetectable amounts).*

Serious injuries, such as head and chest wounds, severe burns, deep cuts that can cause heavy loss of blood and bone fractures, require immediate medical attention. If you are in any doubt as to the nature or seriousness of an injury, always consult a doctor or dial 999 for an ambulance. In addition, swift and effective first aid can help to ease pain and reduce the risk of shock, and may save the casualty's life.

With all serious injuries, the first priority is to prevent further loss of blood and to guard against infection. First-aid treatment carried out as early as possible also helps the body to begin the repair process and so relieve pain.

A first-aid cabinet should be kept fully stocked with equipment such as bandages, sticking plasters and antiseptic wipes, for emergencies and for minor injuries. As well as conventional equipment, however, it's a good idea to keep a variety of household and natural remedies to hand to provide additional relief for a range of injuries.

### NATURE'S FIRST-AID REMEDIES
Many natural remedies that can ease the pain of superficial skin wounds can be found in a well-stocked kitchen or garden. Often simple remedies can hasten healing and prevent infection with the added benefit of few, if any, side effects. Olive oil, for instance, is effective at reducing the inflammation caused by bruising and can be used straight from the bottle.

Other remedies may need to be prepared in advance so they are ready for use when needed. For example, the mashed heads of young marigolds (calendula) preserved in alcohol (vodka is best due to its relative purity) makes an excellent tincture for relieving insect stings. Most kitchens have some or all of the following common ingredients which should form the basis of a natural first-aid chest: butter, salt, sugar, honey, cucumber, apple, onion, potato, cabbage, fresh parsley, garlic, natural yoghurt, red wine vinegar, cider vinegar, tea bags, skimmed milk, cornflour, oatmeal, cayenne pepper, castor oil, safflower oil, olive oil, lemon juice, glycerine, alcohol, bicarbonate of soda, papain (found in meat tenderiser) and ammonia.

With a little planning, your garden can also be a rich source of natural remedies. Skullcap (mad dog weed), valerian root, St John's wort (hypericum), juniper, lavender, burdock, comfrey, marigold, geranium, basil and chickweed can all be beneficial for alleviating pain resulting from superficial injuries such as grazes and burns.

It is also useful to keep a selection of herbal or aromatherapy essential oils to hand for easing pain, encouraging tissue renewal and helping to guard against infection. Basic essential oils include aloe vera, tea tree oil, myrrh, calendula, lavender, vitamin E oil, witch hazel, hyssop, juniper, geranium and eucalyptus (see page 79).

Finally, certain homeopathic remedies such as cantharis, aconite, ledum and arnica can also be kept in your natural remedy first-aid chest. These remedies have various properties that are useful in accident situations, such as alleviating bruising and inflammation, or relieving stress. They will not interfere with the body's normal healing processes or affect any orthodox treatments that may be necessary.

The following pages explain how to use these items for the first-aid treatment of a range of common injuries.

## NATURE'S FIRST-AID CHEST

Keep a stock of natural remedies close at hand so you have ready access to a range of effective treatments for minor household injuries and ailments.

Many items, such as honey, olive oil, cornflour and vinegar, are not only just as effective as comparable manufactured products – they are often more economical too. You should make a list of the items you are using for first-aid purposes and note where they are being stored so you will be able to find them quickly when the need arises.

Check all the items regularly to ensure you have an adequate supply in case of emergency, and replace anything that has passed its best-before date or is showing signs of degenerating.

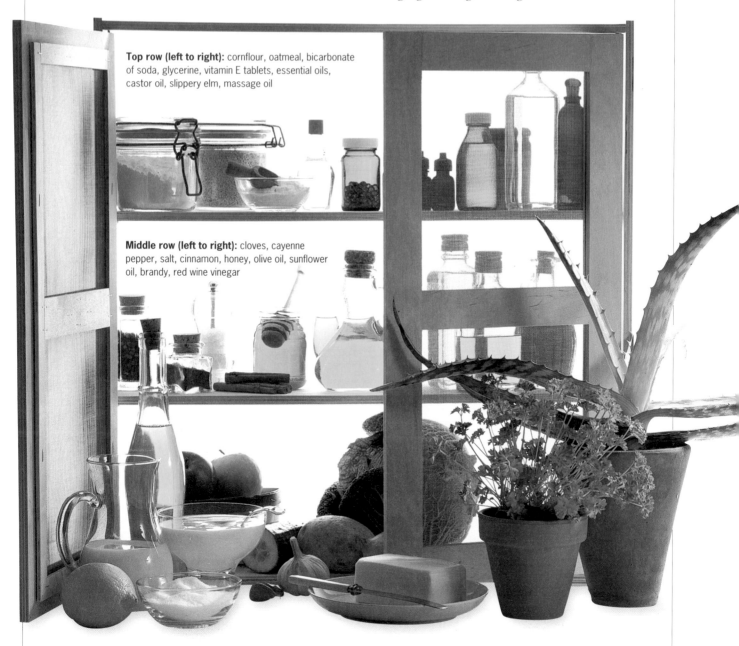

**Top row (left to right):** cornflour, oatmeal, bicarbonate of soda, glycerine, vitamin E tablets, essential oils, castor oil, slippery elm, massage oil

**Middle row (left to right):** cloves, cayenne pepper, salt, cinnamon, honey, olive oil, sunflower oil, brandy, red wine vinegar

**Bottom row (left to right):** lemon, milk, sugar, yoghurt, cider vinegar, apples, cucumber, garlic, potato, cabbage, butter, parsley, aloe vera

*SAFE STORAGE*
*Make sure that natural products for use in first aid are as fresh as possible. Keep highly perishable items, such as dairy products, in the refrigerator and store other items in a cool, dark cupboard where they will be safe from insects and other pests.*

# Injuries to Skin

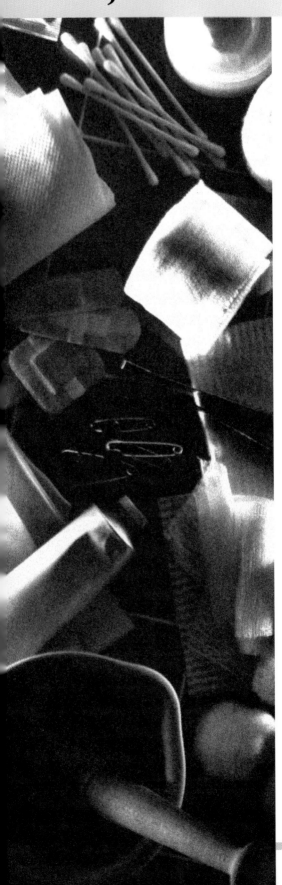

*The skin is well supplied with nerve endings which alert the brain immediately to any injury. Pain from a wound indicates that there may be a loss of blood and a risk of infection, so urgent attention to the injury is required.*

The skin is a versatile protective cover for the body. It is waterproof, supple and sensitive, and capable of stretching to accommodate the movement of the body. The skin plays a vital role in retaining bodily fluids and keeping infection out.

To function efficiently the skin must be kept supple and healthy. Excessive washing of the face and hands, especially in cold weather, can make the skin rough and sore. As the natural oils that keep the skin supple are washed away, the skin dries out and can crack. This common condition, called chapping, can be avoided by using a barrier cream and making sure your hands and face are thoroughly dry after washing them. Regular use of a lanolin-based hand or face cream, moisturiser or bath oil will minimise further chafing and the pain associated with chapped hands.

If a skin condition is no better after two weeks of self-treatment, it may indicate a condition such as eczema or psoriasis, in which case you should see your doctor who may refer you to a specialist. If the skin becomes damaged it must be protected with a dressing such as a sticking plaster, clean gauze or bandage, depending on the wound.

## TREATMENT FOR SHOCK

After injury, blood pressure may drop, leading to potentially fatal shock. Look for warning signs such as pale, cold, clammy skin, rapid, shallow breathing, dizziness, shivering and sweating.

*FIRST AID FOR SHOCK*
*Lay the injured person down on his or her side and check that the casualty can breathe easily. Loosen any tight clothing around the waist, chest and neck and keep the casualty warm by covering with a coat or blanket. Seek medical help immediately.*

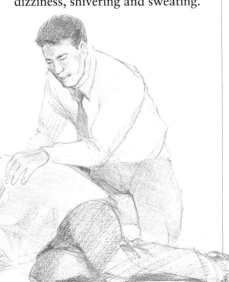

## MINOR CUTS AND GRAZES

Children in particular are prone to minor cuts and grazes. Grazes are less serious than cuts because damage is superficial and there is little loss of blood. However, they are often more painful because layers of skin have been removed over a wider area, exposing more sensitive nerve endings. Minor cuts only involve damage to the small blood vessels near the surface of the skin known as capillaries, and although they may bleed profusely at first the bleeding soon stops. However, cuts and grazes can both become very painful if infected, and thorough cleaning and disinfecting of the wound is extremely important.

### Natural treatment for cuts

There are a variety of natural remedies that help to heal minor cuts and grazes. Tea tree oil is a natural antiseptic – add a few drops to the water you use to wash the wound. Aloe vera can be applied directly onto the wound as a gel or a concentrated liquid. It is a natural antibiotic and also relieves the pain. You should then bandage the wound with a sterile dressing. To promote healing, add calendula cream or comfrey oil to the bandage. A few drops can be mixed into the water you use to wash the wound.

Plain granulated sugar or honey accelerates healing, soothes pain and helps to prevent scarring. It can be packed onto a cleaned cut or wound and then covered with gauze, but make sure the wound has stopped bleeding, or the sugar can make the bleeding worse.

When dressing a cut, you can add any of the following to the bandage or gauze to promote healing:

▸ *A tincture of myrrh, consisting of one part myrrh to six parts water, acts as a natural antiseptic.*

▸ *A tincture of calendula.*

▸ *Comfrey oil or an infusion of the herb.*

▸ *Gel squeezed from the leaf of an aloe vera plant (see right).*

---

### ✚ For minor skin wounds

▪Rinse the injured area under cold running water to wash the wound and slow or stop the bleeding.

▪Gently remove any debris, such as gravel or glass splinters, using cottonwool swabs, gauze or tweezers.

▪Clean with antiseptic wipes, or use gauze or cottonwool swabs dipped in a mild antiseptic. Once it is clean, dab the injured area dry and then cover it with a plaster or a dressing held in place with a bandage.

---

### USING ALOE VERA

Grow your own aloe vera plant for a ready source of fresh gel to apply to cuts and bruises.

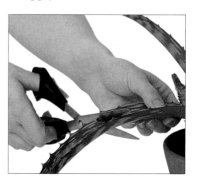

1 *With a pair of scissors, snip off a large leaf; using a sharp blade, cut a slit along its length.*

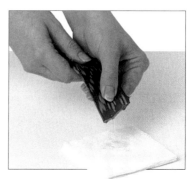

2 *Open out the leaf and squeeze the contents onto a moistened, absorbent cloth. Place over the cut.*

---

## BRUISES

Any blow to the body that damages the capillaries under the skin will cause bruising as blood leaks into the tissues. Most bruises are not serious but can still be painful. Heavy bruising to the face, head, chest, back or abdomen could indicate internal injuries and should be examined by a doctor.

### Natural treatment for bruises

There are several natural remedies that can reduce the pain and swelling of bruises, such as bathing the injury with herbal witch hazel skin toner or applying arnica or comfrey ointment (if the skin is not broken). A cold compress soaked in a lavender infusion is also effective. Honey or vegetable oils like castor, olive or safflower, mixed together or individually, are natural remedies that can ease the pain of a bruise. Spread over the bruised area several times a day or take 3 ml by mouth twice daily. Similarly, cornflour mixed with water or vegetable oil applied externally will relieve pain, as will a tea of St John's wort.

---

### ✚ For bruises

▪You can ease the pain of bruising with a cold compress: soak a cloth in cold water, then wring out and apply to the bruised area for 10 minutes. This restricts the internal bleeding and reduces swelling. Or you can make an ice pack by wrapping a packet of frozen peas in a towel: do not leave an ice pack in contact with the bruise for longer than 10 minutes.

## SUNBURN

Some cases of sunburn are severe enough to cause blisters, in which case they should be treated like any other minor burn (see below). If you experience chills, nausea, fever, intense itchiness, or feel faint you may be suffering from sunstroke and should seek medical attention as soon as possible.

### Natural treatment for sunburn

Place a cold compress on the burn to reduce inflammation and then apply calamine lotion to soothe the pain. Your kitchen can also provide a wide range of natural remedies to bring relief from the inflammation and pain of sunburn. For example, slices of cucumber, apple, yoghurt, raw potato, cider vinegar, moist tea bags and even compresses soaked in skimmed milk and applied to the face and body are safe, natural and inexpensive treatments. These can be combined with skin moisturisers. Aloe vera, calendula, and witch hazel are also soothing. Adding 5 drops of lavender essential oil to a base such as almond oil and massaging in brings rapid relief. Hypercal cream or lotion (a mixture of hypericum and calendula) can aid rapid healing.

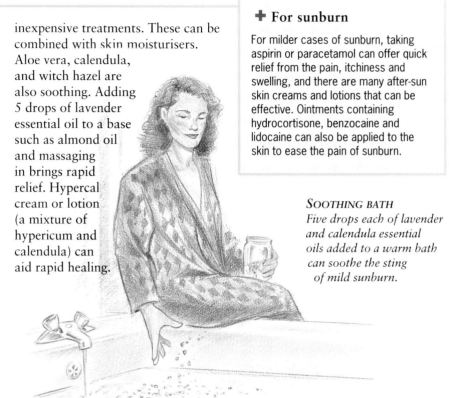

**+ For sunburn**

For milder cases of sunburn, taking aspirin or paracetamol can offer quick relief from the pain, itchiness and swelling, and there are many after-sun skin creams and lotions that can be effective. Ointments containing hydrocortisone, benzocaine and lidocaine can also be applied to the skin to ease the pain of sunburn.

*SOOTHING BATH*
*Five drops each of lavender and calendula essential oils added to a warm bath can soothe the the sting of mild sunburn.*

## MINOR BURNS

Burns to the skin can be caused by a wide range of factors – fire, hot metal, hot liquid, hot vapour, intense cold, electricity, chemicals or the sun. The seriousness of a burn depends upon the area of the body that is affected and the depth to which the skin has been damaged.

In superficial or first degree burns, only the outer layers of skin are damaged, causing soreness, redness and slight swelling. They are most often caused by hot vapour, a hot drink, the sun or by touching a hot saucepan or other hot object. The pain can be reduced by keeping the burn under cold running water for a minimum of 10 minutes.

Seek emergency medical help if the burn affects an extensive area, if the skin is broken, severely blistered or charred, or if the victim is suffering severe pain. Burns on the face or hands may cause scarring and should always be examined by a doctor.

Medical aid is also needed for burns to the eyes, feet, pelvic and pubic areas; any burn where you are not sure of the depth or extent of the injury; and any wound that shows signs of infection or has not healed properly within 10 days.

### Natural treatment for minor burns

After immersing the burn in cold running water, add a few drops of calendula tincture to cold water and apply to the burnt area as a cold compress. After allowing 24 hours for the burn to start the healing process, apply vitamin E oil or lavender oil (4 drops per 60 ml of water) to promote healing. Calendula ointment or aloe vera gel can also soothe the pain of a burn. Homeopathic remedy cantharis 3c taken every hour can provide pain relief. One dose daily of aconite 12c also has a soothing effect.

**+ For burns**

- Cool the burn as quickly as possible by immersing it under cold running water for a minimum of 10 minutes, by covering it with a towel soaked in cold water, or by pouring over the burn any available safe liquid, such as water or milk.

- Don't apply any ointment or cream to a burn for the first 24 hours or burst any blisters that form.

- Remove any watches, belts or jewellery that may constrict the burnt area before it starts to swell. Don't remove any clothing that is stuck to the wound.

- Cover the burn with a clean non-fluffy material such as a sterile dressing or newly laundered handkerchief. You don't need to cover a burn to the face.

- Seek immediate medical attention for any serious burn, especially around the face or pubic areas.

## BLISTERS

A blister is a pocket of fluid that forms under the skin. In addition to burns, a common cause of blisters is friction, for example, as a result of wearing new or badly fitting shoes. If the blister becomes inflamed, swollen and painful, or exudes a cloudy or unpleasant smelling fluid it may have become infected, in which case you should see a doctor.

### Natural treatment for blisters

Natural pain-relieving remedies include a cornflour poultice and vegetable oil lightly applied to the blister before bandaging. Aloe vera gel or the liquid from a capsule of vitamin A or E applied to the blister can help soothe the pain and hasten healing. Lavender essential oil is also effective when dabbed on the blister.

### + For blisters

■ Avoid bursting a blister, if possible, as this increases the risk of infection. If the blister is likely to burst, however, wash the area with soap and a mild disinfectant and then carefully puncture it with a sterilised needle or blade and cover with a sterile dressing. Avoid getting the dressing wet.

## STINGS AND BITES

Insect stings are rarely dangerous unless the victim has had multiple stings, or is allergic to stings, or the stings are around the mouth or throat, which can cause swelling that may obstruct breathing. Jellyfish and corals can also cause painful stings.

### Natural treatment for stings and bites

Once the sting has been removed and the area cleaned, the alkaline sting of an ant or wasp can be eased with lemon juice or vinegar.

Bee stings are acidic so use bicarbonate of soda, washing blue, ammonia, or the papain in meat tenderiser (used in barbecue cooking). Cider vinegar and garlic are natural antiseptics while raw onion draws out the poison. For bee or wasp stings take homeopathic wild rosemary 6c.

For insect bites, a pulped fresh marigold flower can be applied to the wound and bandaged in place to encourage healing. A warm moist compress of burdock also helps to heal the wound. Butter, applied directly, or salt, moistened slightly with water, are natural antiseptics.

For jellyfish stings pour vinegar or alcohol over the injured area to deactivate any stings remaining in the skin. These can then be removed with adhesive tape. Calamine lotion spread over the injured area will help to ease the pain and inflammation.

### STINGER OR BITER?

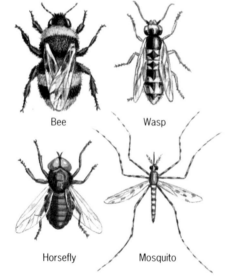

Bee    Wasp

Horsefly    Mosquito

*AIRBORNE ATTACK*
*Stinging insects such as bees and wasps inject poison under the skin. Biting insects such as mosquitoes and horseflies break through the skin to draw up blood.*

### + For stings

■ If the sting has been left behind in the flesh, you must remove it as quickly as possible using your nail, a needle, a pair of tweezers or brushing it out with a card.

■ Try to avoid squeezing the poison sac which constitutes the sting, as this may release more poison into the bloodstream.

■ Hydrocortisone cream or a cold compress applied to the injury will reduce swelling. If the injury is in or around the mouth or throat, give the casualty ice to suck and phone 999 for an ambulance.

■ If the casualty feels unwell or has difficulty breathing, they may be suffering anaphylactic shock, a life-threatening allergic reaction to the sting (see page 150). Keep the casualty calm, loosen restricting clothing, especially around the neck, and phone 999 for an ambulance.

### STING AND BITE PREVENTION

There are many ways to prevent insect bites and stings. Food supplements vitamin $B_1$, zinc and garlic are all released through the skin in tiny amounts and repel insects. Other natural repellents include 5 drops of eucalyptus or citronella oils added to a cup of water and applied to exposed areas of skin. Cider vinegar is also effective. Dark clothes attract insects, so wear light clothes, especially in the evening, and keep wrists, arms and legs covered. Place insect screens over windows and, in tropical countries, sleep under a mosquito net that has been sprayed with insecticide.

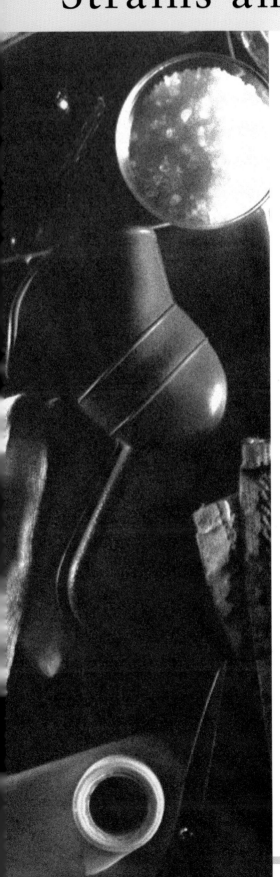

# Strains and Sprains

*It is helpful to learn how to distinguish the different types of musculoskeletal injury, such as strains, sprains or fractures. Many types of injury can be treated at home using simple first aid measures, while others may need expert medical attention.*

Sport, accidental injury, and poor exercise technique (for example, if not fully warmed up) can result in damage to muscles and other soft tissues, particularly around a joint. Ligaments, tendons and muscles may be twisted or torn, bones may be broken (fractured) or dislocated.

Joint strains and sprains usually cause pain and swelling and restricted movement in the limb. In many cases, these injuries may be treated safely at home with a combination of conventional and natural therapies.

Serious limb fractures can often be identified by sight, for example if the limb is badly swollen or hanging at an unusual angle, or (in the case of compound fractures) if the bone protrudes through the skin.

Movement will be difficult or impossible and pain can be throbbing, shooting, stabbing, aching or unbearably sharp. In these cases, movement must be prevented to avoid further damage.

It can often be difficult to tell the difference between the various types of musculoskeletal damage. If in any doubt about the severity of an injury, treat as a suspected fracture, provide support for the injured limb and arrange transport to hospital.

## STRAIN OR SPRAIN?

A sprain is damage to a ligament at or near a joint, whereas a strain is damage to a muscle. One way to identify the injury is to note which movements cause the most pain. Ask someone to bend the limb for you without you making any effort. If it still hurts or is restricted, the problem is a joint injury (sprain). If it no longer hurts, or is restricted when someone tries to straighten it, it is a muscle injury (strain).

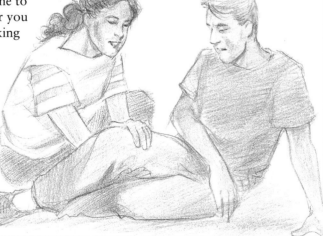

*KNEE INJURY*
*The pain of a knee injury may stem from the joint itself or from soft tissues around it.*

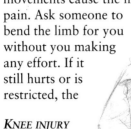

# CRAMPS

A cramp is a painful muscle spasm caused by a sudden excessive contraction of the muscle fibres. They are usually involuntary, strike unexpectedly and can be quite crippling temporarily. Often they occur at night and affect the calf muscle, particularly after a day of unaccustomed exercise which produces a build up of lactic acid in the muscles. They can also be caused by repetitive actions, poor circulation, sitting in an awkward position, or swimming in cold water.

Muscle cramps are common during or after exercise, due to excessive loss of salt and body fluids from sweating. Replenishing these fluids with electrolytic sports drinks during exercise can help to prevent the problem. Cramps may sometimes occur if the muscles are cold when starting exercise. You can avoid this problem by going through a planned warm-up routine before exercising.

Strenuous physical activity carried out too soon after eating a big meal can also lead to cramp because the blood supply is diverted to the digestive system and there is insufficient blood reaching the muscles. Always wait at least one hour after eating before exercising.

## Natural treatment to prevent muscle cramps

Ensure your diet contains an adequate supply of vitamin D and calcium (see page 58) to reduce the risk of muscle spasms. Vitamin E supplements have also been shown to help avoid night cramps.

Hot and cold compresses can improve circulation to the affected muscles, and a mustard foot bath may help to relieve leg cramps.

Basil, marjoram and lemon grass essential oils added to a warm bath or mixed with a base oil and massaged into the muscles can help to alleviate the problem of recurring cramps.

## ✚ For muscle cramps

- A good way of forcing a muscle with cramp to relax is to try stretching the muscle out again.

- If you have calf cramps, you can stimulate the blood circulation to the muscle by massaging the leg in upwards movements towards the heart. This helps to flush out lactic acid and prevent the muscles becoming stiff again later.

- A hot shower will help to improve circulation and bring further relief.

*FIGHTING MUSCLE CRAMPS*
*This exercise can help to avoid cramp in the calf muscles: stand about 1 m (3 ft) away from a wall, with your feet flat on the floor and legs straight. Lean towards the wall and press against it with your palms. Stretch and hold for 10 seconds. Repeat several times.*

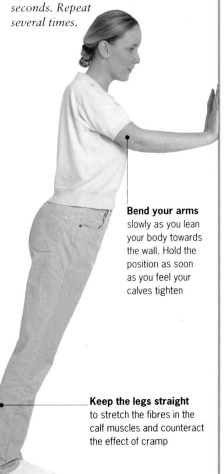

**Bend your arms** slowly as you lean your body towards the wall. Hold the position as soon as you feel your calves tighten

**Keep the legs straight** to stretch the fibres in the calf muscles and counteract the effect of cramp

## MAKING A COMPRESS

A cold compress can be used to treat bruising and minor strain and sprain injuries. It is a good way to reduce inflammation, swelling and bleeding under the skin and to soothe pain. An ice pack is effective for reducing swelling in serious joint injuries. To make an ice pack, fill a plastic bag with crushed or cubed ice (or use a bag of frozen peas). Wrap the ice pack in a towel and apply to the injury. Repeat as necessary. Never apply ice directly to the skin as this causes ice burns. A hot compress is used to improve circulation and aid healing.

1 *Take a piece of non-fluffy cloth or cotton wool and soak in cold water. The cloth should be sterile, even if the skin is unbroken, as in the case of a bruise or sprain.*

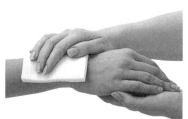

2 *Squeeze or wring out the cloth so that it is damp but not dripping, and place it firmly on the injured area.*

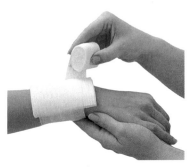

3 *Replace the compress with a fresh one regularly so that the cooling effect is maintained. If necessary, hold the compress in place with an open weave bandage.*

## STRAINS AND SPRAINS

All joints are vulnerable to strains and sprains, especially resulting from accidental falls and injuries sustained in contact sports such as football.

The knee is particularly prone to damage because it is made up of a complex arrangement of cartilage, ligaments, muscles, tendons and bones which must allow movement and support the weight of the body (see below). If any of these structures are damaged the effect can be painful and the knee may stiffen or be unable to support the weight of the individual. The pain of a strained or sprained knee is described as sharp, intense, stabbing or tender.

A sprained ankle is a painful injury involving any one of a number of ligaments and tendons at different sites on the joint. The ligament at the top of the foot is the most vulnerable to injury. If you trip and put your weight heavily on one foot, this ligament absorbs most of the impact and can be damaged. This type of injury can take a long time to heal because the ligaments have a poor blood supply. Treatment aims to rest the injury to aid healing and to reduce pain and swelling.

### Natural treatment

Once first aid has been applied (see box, right) a number of natural therapies can help to reduce the pain.

---

### ✚ For sprained joints

■ Rest the injured part by supporting the limb in a comfortable position.

■ Ice should be applied every 20 minutes for a few hours to reduce pain, swelling and bruising. This treatment should be repeated four or five times over the first 24 hours.

■ Compress the injured joint by padding with cotton wool or plastic foam and securing with a roller bandage. You can compress and chill the injured area at the same time by using a roller bandage to hold an ice pack in position.

■ Elevate and support the limb to reduce blood flow to the joint and thus reduce swelling and bruising.

---

Lightly massaging the injury will help to improve circulation and drain any fluid that has built up. Comfrey leaves applied as a poultice can aid the repair of tissue and cartilage. To use, bruise the leaves and wrap in a dressing. Avoid placing the leaves directly on the skin as they may cause irritation.

The homeopathic remedy Arnica mother tincture, added to water, can be applied on a moist compress to reduce swelling. Rhus tox or Ruta graveolens can assist the long-term repair of ligaments and tendons, while Ledum can ease the pain.

---

### FIGURE OF EIGHT BANDAGING

Bandages must be wide enough to cover the wound and extend 2.5 cm (1 in) beyond it. Ensure the bandage is firm but not too tight. Check regularly and adjust as necessary.

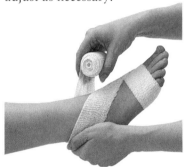

*1 Holding the foot with one hand, wind the bandage once around the top of the foot, working from the inside outwards. Make sure that the bandage is not too tight.*

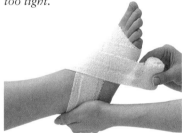

*2 Wind the bandage from the inside of the ankle across the foot to the little toe. Take it under the foot and then up by the big toe. Now take it under the foot again.*

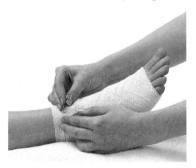

*3 Wind the bandage across the top of the foot and behind the ankle in a figure of eight pattern. Continue until the foot is covered. Wind around the ankle and secure.*

---

*THE KNEE JOINT*
*The knee joint is lined with smooth pads of cartilage (menisci) and cushioned by fluid-filled sacs (bursas). The knee tendons link the tibia, a bone in the lower leg, with the quadriceps muscle. Ligaments add support. The knee is an unusual joint in that a special bone, the knee cap or patella, is incorporated in the tendons to add protection. The knee is vulnerable to injuries such as torn or sprained cartilage, tendon, muscle and ligaments; dislocated patella and inflamed bursa (bursitis).*

Tendon
Patella
Ligament
Tendon
Ligament
Meniscus

# INDEX

# ACKNOWLEDGMENTS

**Carroll & Brown Limited**
would like to thank
Sharon Freed
Madeleine Jennings
Trish Shine

**Editorial assistance**
Jennifer Mussett

**Design assistance**
Rachel Goldsmith

**Photograph sources**
8 Wellcome Institute Library, London
9 (Top) Mary Evans Picture Library; (Bottom) Carroll & Brown Ltd
11 Alvis Upitis/Image Bank
12 Zefa
17 Professor P.M. Motta/ University 'La Sapienza', Rome/ Science Photo Library
19 Matt Meadows/Peter Arnold Inc/Science Photo Library
25 Kobal Collection
26 Boston Medical Library, in The Francis A. Countway Library of Medicine, Boston, Mass, USA
28 Kobal Collection
29 (Top) Angela Hampton/ Family Life Pictures; (Centre) J. Wakelin/Trip; (Bottom) Frank Schneidermeyer/ Oxford Scientific Films

34 Zefa
36 Kobal Collection
38 Eye of Science/Science Photo Library
42 Wellcome Institute Library
47 Deni Bown/Oxford Scientific Films
50 Scott Camazine/Oxford Scientific Films
60 National Back Pain Association
62 S. B. Paul McCullagh/Oxford Scientific Films
66 National Back Pain Association
68 Zefa
71 Science Photo Library
72 David Kirk-Campbell/Rolf Institute of Structural Integration, Boulder, Colorado, USA
73 Simon Fraser, Hexam General Hospital/Science Photo Library
76 The Society of Teachers of the Alexander Technique
106 Marc Romanelli/Image Bank
132 CNRI/Science Photo Library
138 Tony Stone Images
140 (Top) Zefa (Bottom) Gilda Pacitti
146 Photograph courtesy of St Christopher's Hospital
148 Jos Korenromp/Oxford Scientific Films

**Illustrators**
Joanna Cameron
Karen Cochrane
John Geary
Sandie Hill
Christine Pilsworth
Lesli Sternberg
Sarah Venus
Paul Williams

**Photographic assistants**
M. A. Hugo
Mark Langridge

**Hair and make-up**
Kim Menzies

**Picture researcher**
Sandra Schneider

**Research**
Stephen Chong

**Index**
Richard Emerson

75-007-01